BRAIN FOODS *for* KIDS

BRAIN FOODS for KIDS

Over 100 recipes to boost your child's intelligence

NICOLA GRAIMES

DELTA TRADE PAPERBACKS

Delta
Trade Paperbacks

BRAIN FOODS FOR KIDS
Over 100 Recipes to Boost Your Child's Intelligence
A Delta Book

PUBLISHING HISTORY
Carroll & Brown edition published in 2004
Delta trade paperback edition / March 2005

Published by
Bantam Dell
A Division of Random House, Inc.
New York, New York

Project Editor: Caroline Smith
Art Editor: Anne Fisher
Photographer: Jules Selmes

Library of Congress Cataloging in Publication Data
Graimes, Nicola
Brain foods for kids : over 100 recipes to boost your child's intelligence / Nicola Graimes.
p. cm.
Includes index.
ISBN 0-553-38335-3
1. Children--Nutrition. 2. Intellect--Nutritional aspects. 3. Nootropic agents.
RJ206.G59 2005
613.2'083--dc22   2004051268

Printed and bound by Everbest in Hong Kong, China.
Published simultaneously in Canada

www.bantamdell.com

10 9 8 7 6 5 4 3 2 1

CONTENTS

INTRODUCTION

All our children come into this world with a certain amount of intelligence. Yet, the question that fascinates me and has spurred me to research and write this book is – can we, as parents, help our children improve on their inherent intelligence through a healthy diet and lifestyle?

From birth, children are constantly learning new skills, from the first smile to talking, from crawling to walking and running, then on to reading and writing. Their brains need constant, good-quality nourishment to perform these functions and a whole range of other tasks. To put it into perspective, the brain represents just two percent of body weight but demands a massive 30 percent of the body's total energy supply.

My interest in child intelligence and behavior has been further fueled by the growing scientific evidence that you can enhance your child's brain-power by providing him or her with certain nutrients and that a deficiency in just one nutrient may have a detrimental effect on behavior and learning capabilities.

Now, this may sound straightforward, but as we all know, children can be very fickle in their tastes and eating habits. Most parents have their own methods of getting their children to eat. Mine are probably no different from many others. I know that it's best not to panic, to avoid confrontation at mealtimes, and to avoid giving children "junk" in place of decent meals just because they won't eat what you've given them. I've also realized that with a little gentle persuasion and by providing children with as much variety as possible, you'll be on the right track. My daughter went through some very fussy food fads: in her eyes she had better things to do than sit down and eat a meal. But now, happily, the tables have turned and she eats most things that are put in front of her. My son seemed to be following suit, but now, rather than preparing an endless collection of dishes in the hope that he will eat something, I've relaxed, and know that he will eat if he's hungry.

Parents have a lot to contend with. Children are influenced by TV advertising for highly colored drinks, fast food, and processed snacks, by peer pressure, and by the lure of the free toys offered by some manufacturers. The statistics are frightening: more children than ever are overweight (just look around the playground) and are therefore at greater risk of life-threatening conditions such as heart disease and diabetes. What's more, the social stigma of being overweight can have a seriously detrimental effect on a child's confidence.

We all want the best for our children and providing them with a good, balanced diet gives them the best start in life. The following recommendations are at the heart of this book.

YOUR BRAINBOOSTING ACTION PLAN

Eating the right foods and cutting out the junk is the crucial first step toward providing the brain with the nutrients it needs for normal brain function.

The power of exercise *One recent study showed that 40 to 69 percent of children are largely inactive – yet physical exercise is fundamentally important in nurturing both body and mind. Running, swimming, and other aerobic exercise increases the supply of oxygenated blood to the brain, benefiting memory and attention span.*

A good start *Research has found that eating breakfast is the best way to get brain cells fired up, improving memory and concentration. A good mix of protein and carbohydrates is recommended. See page 41.*

Little and often *Children have high energy requirements relative to their size, so they need energy-dense, nutritious foods in small but regular amounts. Regular meals and healthy snacks will keep blood sugar levels steady and ensure sustained amounts of energy. See page 42.*

Fresh is best *Fruits and vegetables are crucial for good health and well-being and are great sources of vital antioxidant vitamins and minerals for the brain. However, recent research has shown that children eat less than half the recommended five portions of fruits and vegetables a day. See page 20.*

Fishy business *Studies confirm that consuming fish oils can raise IQ levels even before birth and they have also been shown to benefit children with dyslexia and ADHD. See page 18.*

Dump the junk *Poor-quality, high-fat, high-sugar, additive-laden foods do no one any favors, unsettling blood sugar levels and robbing the body of vital nutrients. See page 27.*

Role of iron *Studies have shown a positive link between IQ scores and iron intake, yet iron deficiency is common. Lack of iron is associated with delays in development, poor concentration, irritability, mood swings, and depression. See page 17.*

Water for life *Most children don't drink enough water, favoring cans of carbonated drinks instead. Dehydration can affect concentration and intellectual performance, as well as the transportation of nutrients around the body. See page 23.*

Building
A BETTER BRAIN

Here you'll find a wealth of advice about how to enhance your child's brainpower. Individual beneficial nutrients are mentioned, but it is important to recognize that any one of these should form part of an overall balanced diet and active lifestyle. The hope is that you will take on board many of the suggestions found here: long-term improvements in diet should start with our children – and the younger the better.

Bright BEGINNINGS

From the moment of conception, your child needs certain nutrients to help him or her develop healthily. So what you eat during pregnancy is very important in making sure your baby has a healthy brain and body. By including the recommended brain foods in your diet, you can pass on their benefits to your developing baby.

A Healthy Pregnancy Diet

In terms of eating the right food, the first few weeks of pregnancy are some of the most important. However, at this point, many women won't realize that they are pregnant. So if you're planning to have a baby, it's a good idea to start eating a nutrient-rich diet before you conceive. And, if you do miss those early weeks, don't worry. Simply start to eat well once you know you are pregnant.

During the first six months of pregnancy, you shouldn't need more food than usual. What is important is the quality of your diet. Pregnancy is a time to nurture both your baby and yourself. Eat the right foods, rich in the right nutrients, and you'll not only help your baby grow but also help yourself to enjoy a healthy pregnancy and good-quality breast milk once your baby is born.

Choose fresh rather than processed foods whenever possible and eat at least five portions of fruits and vegetables a day for essential vitamins, antioxidants, minerals, and fiber. Try to eat a range of different types and colors of fruits and vegetables for optimum benefit.

Substitute caffeine-free herbal teas and coffee alternatives for the real stuff.

VITAMINS

As your baby begins to grow inside you, the brain is one of his or her first organs to develop. An adequate supply of folic acid, one of the B vitamins, is vital to its healthy development. Folic acid works alongside vitamin B_{12} to form new cells and is crucial to the development of the spinal cord – inadequate supplies may result in neural tube defects, or spina bifida. Therefore, women planning a baby are recommended to take a daily supplement of 400 mcg of folic acid for, ideally, three months before conception and up to the twelfth week of pregnancy. Folic acid can be found in certain foods (see right), so it's also a good idea to add them to your diet to increase your intake. Folic acid is, however, easily destroyed during cooking, so lightly cook vegetables or eat them raw whenever possible.

Vitamin B_{12} is also crucial for the formation of red blood cells. Sources include yeast extract, meat, fish, dairy and soy products, and eggs.

There is new evidence to suggest that vitamins E and C can play a role in reducing the risk of preeclampsia during pregnancy. This rare condition causes a severe rise in blood pressure that is dangerous to both mother and baby. Although most pregnant women won't suffer preeclampsia, it is wise to eat vitamin E–rich foods, such as avocados, sunflower and safflower oils, almonds and hazelnuts, and plenty of fresh fruits and vegetables high in vitamin C. Vitamin C is also important in helping you absorb the iron in your diet – a vital mineral for pregnant women.

MINERALS

During pregnancy, calcium and magnesium are necessary for the developing bones and healthy nervous system of your baby. Your body will absorb calcium more efficiently at this time, but make sure you include adequate amounts of dairy products in your diet. Nondairy sources of calcium and magnesium include soy milk and green leafy vegetables, molasses, sardines, baked beans, and sesame seeds.

Anemia is common in pregnancy, and you need enough iron to create hemoglobin, the part of the red blood cells that carries oxygen to the fetus. For the first six months after birth, babies will absorb iron from breast or formula milk, but they will also rely on iron storage in their bodies – another reason for making sure your iron intake during pregnancy is sufficient. You can get iron from foods such as red meat, dark poultry meat, eggs, leafy green vegetables, dried fruit, fortified breakfast cereals, whole grains, nuts, and legumes.

ESSENTIAL FATTY ACIDS

It is important to include a good range of essential fatty acids in your diet. Oily fish is a good source of the long-chain polyunsaturated fats DHA (docosahexaenoic acid) and EPA (eicosapentaenoic acid), fundamental to healthy eye and brain development. Women should ensure adequate levels prior to conception, throughout pregnancy, and while breastfeeding, since 70 percent of the cells that make up the adult brain are formed before birth. Two portions of fish are recommended per week, one of which should be oily, such as tuna, salmon, sardines, trout, or mackerel.

A Norwegian study looked at the infants of nearly 600 women who were given an

nutrient
KNOW-HOW

GOOD SOURCES OF FOLIC ACID

- Nuts & seeds
- Eggs
- Fortified breakfast cereals, wheat germ, bread & flour
- Legumes & lentils
- Avocados
- Leafy green vegetables, such as spinach, lettuce & other salad greens
- Broccoli, brussels sprouts, & asparagus
- Orange juice

OFF THE MENU

Liver is high in vitamin A, which can damage the developing fetus if eaten in excessive amounts.

Soft and blue-veined cheese such as Brie, Stilton, and Camembert can harbor a bacterium called *Listeria*, which may cause miscarriage or stillbirth.

Peanuts are causing increasingly greater numbers of children to suffer from allergic reactions. It is now believed that sensitivity to peanuts can start in the womb, so it is advisable to cut them out during pregnancy, particularly if there is a history of peanut allergy, hay fever, eczema, or asthma in the family.

Uncooked or partially cooked eggs may harbor salmonella.

Shark, swordfish, and marlin, and more than two medium-size cans of tuna or one fresh tuna steak a week, should be avoided by pregnant and breastfeeding women, and those intending to conceive. This is due to the levels of mercury present in these fish, which can harm an unborn child's nervous system. The US Food and Drug Administration (FDA) also recommends avoiding tilefish and king mackerel for the same reason.

Alcohol depletes zinc levels and can cross the placenta, causing birth defects if drunk in excess. To be on the safe side, cut it out altogether.

Caffeine also can cross the placenta and drinking excessive amounts (more than 6 cups a day) has been linked to nerve abnormalities and low birth weight. Pregnant women are now recommended to limit the amount of caffeine they consume to no more than 300mg a day (see opposite). Caffeine is found in tea, coffee, some carbonated drinks, and chocolate. Tea also interferes with iron absorption.

omega-3 supplement from 18 weeks of pregnancy to three months after birth. Researchers looked at the cognitive performance of the breastfed infants from birth up until age 4 and concluded that the omega-3 supplement seemed to enhance mental development in the children.

Eggs (thoroughly cooked), walnuts, and linseeds also provide omega-3 fatty acids, while the equally vital omega-6, which assists in normal nerve function, is found in other nuts and seeds and their oils.

CHOLINE

To have a good memory, your child's brain needs the neurotransmitter acetylcholine, a deficiency of which is probably the most common cause of memory decline. It is derived from the nutrient choline, which is found particularly in egg yolks, grains, nuts, beans, and fish such as sardines. Vitamins B_1, B_5, B_{12}, and C, as well as lecithin, are also essential for the formation of acetylcholine.

SUPPLEMENTS

If you've suffered from severe morning sickness or if your diet is poor, it may be wise to consider a specially formulated vitamin and mineral supplement for pregnant women. This can give you a good balance of nutrients, including beta-carotene (the plant version of vitamin A, which is not recommended in large amounts), zinc, iron, magnesium, and calcium, which are important for the developing fetus and can help with muscle cramps.

The Early Months

Once your baby is born, there's no doubt that breastfeeding is the best start you can give your child. Your breast milk contains everything your baby needs in just the right quantities. It is rich in protein, minerals (including iron and calcium), and vitamins A, D, and B_{12}. Current recommendations from the World Health Organization advise mothers to feed their babies only breast milk until they are at least six months old. Breast milk also boosts immunity and protects against the risk of gastroenteritis, ear and respiratory infections, asthma, and eczema.

POSTPREGNANCY DIET

Nursing mothers are advised to consume 450 more calories than the average daily recommendation of 2,000 calories, as you will need extra energy and nutrients. However, you will use up some of the storage laid down in pregnancy while breastfeeding, which may go some way toward returning you to a pre-pregnancy weight.The recommendations on the preceding pages should be followed to ensure your baby receives an adequate supply of nutrients, including the essential fatty acids and choline. Some of these substances are naturally present in breast milk but your diet can also play an important role.

BREASTFEEDING AS BRAIN FOOD

Breast milk is vital to the development of your child's brain and central nervous system, as it contains crucial fatty acids including omega-3 and -6, which can positively affect cognitive development. Recent research also shows that breastfeeding can help improve a child's long-term intelligence. Breastfed babies tend to have higher IQs than formula-fed babies. Additionally, new research has shown it may be possible for breastfeeding mothers to permanently enhance the memories of their babies. This is due to the nutrient choline, which is found in breast milk, particularly in the first few days after birth. It is believed that choline is of critical importance in memory development, the determination of adult memory capacity, and resistance to age-related memory impairments.

FORMULA MILK

While it is widely acknowledged that breast milk is the best for a baby's development, formula milk manufacturers have been working hard to improve the nutritional status of their products. It is not always possible for some women to breastfeed, and these mothers should not feel guilty about bottle feeding. Formula milk is made to strict guidelines and manufacturers try to ensure it resembles breast milk as closely as possible. Some are even fortifying milk with the essential fatty acids linked to improving memory and IQ; however, studies suggest that these are not so readily absorbed compared to those in breast milk.

Brain NUTRIENTS

For good health and optimum brain power, a child's diet should contain the "proper" amounts of certain nutrients. Balance and variety are the key, and a deficiency in just one vital nutrient can impair cognitive performance.

nutrient
KNOW-HOW

FIBER

Although essential to keep a mature digestive system working correctly, too many unrefined whole grains and cereals should not be given to children aged under 5. Babies and young children can find fiber difficult to digest in large quantities. They may become full before they have eaten the variety of foods needed for a balanced diet. Instead, offer a balance of refined and unrefined starchy foods.

CARBOHYDRATES

The brain needs a constant and steady supply of glucose, which supplies it with the energy it needs. Carbohydrate foods, and preferably complex carbohydrates, are the best sources, and should make up about a third of a child's diet.

Carbohydrates come in two forms: simple (also known as sugars) and complex (starches). Sugars are either intrinsic, such as those already present in fruit, or extrinsic, such as refined sugar added to sweets, cakes, and cookies.

The carbohydrates in your child's diet should be made up principally of intrinsic sugars and unrefined complex carbohydrates found in whole grain bread, potatoes, legumes, whole wheat pasta, brown rice, and vegetables. Unrefined carbohydrates are preferable to refined because they are higher in nutrients and fiber and, crucially for the brain, they help to keep blood sugar levels steady, providing long-term, sustained energy.

Refined, sugary foods lead to a surge in blood sugar levels, which can be followed by a slump. Your child's concentration and attention span will wane and he or she will become fatigued. Extreme highs and lows in blood sugar levels can result in dizziness, irritability, and mood swings (see also page 26).

PROTEIN

We actually need relatively small amounts of protein (children aged 4–10 need between ½ to one ounce per day), but variety is important to get the full spectrum of the different nutrients found in protein foods. Protein is found in both animal (meat, poultry, eggs, and dairy products) and plant sources (beans, lentils, nuts, and seeds).

Protein is made up of 25 amino acids. Eight of these are known as essential amino acids because they have to be provided by diet and are not made in the body. Among their many roles, amino acids are crucial for making neurotransmitters, the brain's messengers, and so are vital to brain chemistry and emotions. The amino acid tyrosine, found in fish, dairy products, eggs, oats, and turkey can lift mood and increase alertness, while another amino acid, phenylalanine, is used to regulate blood sugar through insulin.

Proteins are said to satisfy the appetite for longer periods than carbohydrates, yet the latter are believed to provide long-term energy. Many foods are a combination of the two.

FAT

The brain is composed of 60 percent fat, which has to come from the diet. The type of fat your child eats, therefore, affects the composition of the fats in his or her brain. This is why it is so important to include the "right" types of fat in your child's diet, as these are essential for brain development and enable children to think and to store and retrieve memories.

Did you know?

SIGNS OF FATTY-ACID DEFICIENCY

- Excessive thirst
- Frequent urination
- Dry skin and hair
- Soft, brittle nails
- Dandruff
- Rough, hard skin on arms and legs
- Behavioral problems
- Learning difficulties
- Hyperactivity
- Poor concentration and memory
- Poor vision

The most useful group of fats for brain and eye function are the long-chain polyunsaturated fatty acids, including omega-3 fats EPA and DHA, but these are also the ones children (and adults) are least likely to get from their diets. A deficiency in omega-3 is said to be one of the major causes of degenerative disease and of a corresponding decline in brain function. There also appears to be a correlation between fatty acid levels in infants and their intellectual and behavioral performance as children.

You will find the richest amounts of omega-3 in oily fish (see page 18) It also is found in eggs and some plant foods, however, these omega-3s are not as potent as those found in fish oils.

The other essential fatty acid is omega-6, found in plant sources such as nuts and seeds,

Did you know?

MULTIVITAMIN AND MINERAL SUPPLEMENTS

There are numerous studies to show that intelligence, especially nonverbal, improves when children are given a multi-vitamin and mineral supplement. However, the general view is that supplements are most effective when a child's diet is poor. If a child follows a healthy and balanced diet, the effects are not so apparent.

Supplements should never be viewed as a replacement for a good diet, but the chances are fairly likely that a typical child eating a typical diet will experience subtle deficiencies in key nutrients at some stage in his or her life. Many manufacturers have come up with multivitamin and mineral supplements specifically for children, and these are the safest bet for parents, since the nutrients are carefully balanced and in the recommended daily amounts. It also is possible to buy essential fatty acid blends (containing omega-3 and -6) for children either in oil or capsule form if you feel your child could be lacking in these.

as well as corn, safflower, and sunflower oils. Phospholipids, other fatty-acid substances found particularly in eggs, fish, and soybeans, are needed for brain cell membrane repair and the transmission of electrical nerve impulses.

Bad fats include saturated as well as hydrogenated or trans fats, which have a negative effect on the brain. Once the hydrogenated fat gets into the cell walls, it interferes with the assimilation of nutrients, resulting in toxic buildup. Unfortunately, it is very easy for children to eat too many "bad" fats, especially if their diets are made up mainly of highly processed or fast foods. Hydrogenated fat is found in a wide range of manufactured foods, from margarine, sausages, and salad dressings to pies, cookies, and cakes. Fortunately, some major food producers are attempting to reduce (or even eliminate) the hydrogenated fat content of their products.

VITAMINS & MINERALS

Brain function is influenced by a variety of essential vitamins and minerals, and pound for pound a child needs a lot more than the average adult. Vitamins and minerals are also crucial for the production of energy, boosting the immune system, the nervous system, and practically every body process.

Vitamins A, C, and E are antioxidants that protect the brain and body from toxins and pollution. Vitamin C is essential for a healthy immune system and for turning food into mental and physical energy. It also helps us to absorb iron.

B vitamins are vital for brain function, a healthy nervous system, and energy metabolism. They are important in the production of the brain neurotransmitters (messengers) dopamine, adrenaline, noradrenaline, and serotonin. Poor concentration and memory, lack of energy, insomnia, and irritability are signs of possible deficiency.

Calcium and magnesium are known as nature's tranquilizers, since they relax nerve and muscle cells. A lack of these minerals can make children feel nervous, irritable, and aggressive. A deficiency of choline, a vitamin-like compound, has been linked to possible memory and thought impairment. Along with lecithin and the B vitamins, choline enables the body to produce acetylcholine, which transmits electrical impulses to the brain and nervous system. Zinc is crucial for memory and brain function. It is also said to be important in the synthesis of the brain-calming chemical serotonin. Boron has been found to aid memory and improve attention and mental alertness and is essential for energy metabolism.

Iron has many functions in the body, one of which is to carry oxygen in the blood. Deficiency can make children feel tired and irritable and less able to concentrate, as well as affecting their development. Numerous studies have found that there are a great number of children (and adults) throughout the world lacking in this vital brain nutrient. Increasing iron consumption can lift mood and reduce anger, while an American study has linked higher intake of iron with a reduction in depression in teenage girls.

Research has also been conducted to see if there is a link between iron in the diet and IQ, and some of these studies have shown a possible positive link between IQ scores and iron intake. Iron from animal sources is better absorbed than that from plant sources, but drinking a glass of orange juice with an iron-rich meal will help to encourage absorption.

Selenium is a powerful antioxidant that can protect the brain from heavy metals such as lead, used in pipes, and mercury, part of the amalgam used in dental fillings. Even small amounts of heavy metals can accumulate in the tissues and interfere with brain chemistry. Chromium helps in the control of blood glucose levels.

VITAL VITAMINS & MINERALS, AND WHERE TO FIND THEM

Vitamin E *Nuts and seeds and their oils*

Vitamin A *Animal foods including dairy, meat, fish, and eggs (as retinol) and in fruit and vegetables (as beta carotene)*

Vitamin C *Kiwi and citrus fruit, berries, green vegetables, tomatoes, and bell peppers*

B vitamins *Whole grains, eggs, green vegetables, brown rice, meat, fish, legumes, nuts and seeds*

Calcium *Dairy products, almonds, apricots, seeds, sardines, and green leafy vegetables*

Magnesium *Soybeans, whole grains, nuts, dried fruit, green leafy vegetables, and meat*

Choline *Egg yolk, sardines, liver, nuts, legumes, and grains*

Zinc *Dark turkey meat, shellfish, beans, and whole grains*

Boron *Nuts, apples, broccoli, peas, grapes, and legumes*

Iron *Red meat, molasses, cocoa, parsley, eggs, legumes, green vegetables, liver, shellfish, and fortified breakfast cereals*

Selenium *Whole grains, cereals, tuna, shellfish, liver, dairy products, and eggs*

Chromium *Red meat, eggs, cheese, seafood, whole grains*

Brain FOODS

Your child's mind needs nurturing and nourishment like any other part of his or her body. Just as a good diet helps maintain a healthy heart, lungs, and digestion, so it can influence the efficiency of the brain's chemical processes, improving memory, concentration, and mental energy. While there are some foods that can be accused of being bad for brain function (see Brain Drain, page 26), there are many that can help children maximize their learning capability.

nutrient
KNOW-HOW

GOOD SOURCES OF OMEGA-3

- Mackerel
- Tuna
- Sardines
- Herring
- Salmon (preferably wild or organic)
- Anchovies
- Trout
- Sturgeon
- Small amounts in white fish and shellfish

NONFISH SOURCES
- Walnuts
- Linseeds (or flaxseed)
- Pumpkin seeds
- Eggs
- Soybeans

FISH & SHELLFISH

It is now widely recognized that fish and shellfish are great brain food – it's not just an old wives' tale! They contain the beneficial essential fatty acid omega-3, along with other vitamins, minerals, and amino acids. Found in the richest amounts in oily fish, omega-3 fatty acids DHA and EPA have been shown to be essential for the health and development of nerves, eyes, and brain function. (The old favorite, cod-liver oil, is not the best source of essential oils for children, since any pollutants tend to be stored in a fish's liver.)

These fatty acids are not produced in the body and so have to be supplied by diet. There is widespread concern that modern diets do not contain enough omega-3 fats, a lack of which

Wonder food?

FISH- AND PLANT-OIL SUPPLEMENTS

A recent study in the UK found that giving children fish- and plant-oil supplements over a three-month period had impressive results. A group of teachers was asked to select children who had shown slight difficulties in learning, memory, and concentration. Half were given the supplements and the other half a placebo. Over 40 percent of those taking the supplements improved their scores in intelligence tests and demonstrated improvements in reading age and numeracy. Research also shows that the Japanese, who eat a lot of fish, have, on average, IQs 6 percent higher than the average American.

has been linked to poor concentration and memory, dyslexia, behavioral problems, and learning difficulties as well as hyperactivity in some sensitive children.

Children particularly need omega-3 fatty acids for their rapidly developing brains, eyes, and nerves. Omega-3 has also been shown to improve mood and can help with feelings of depression. One serving of oily fish a week is recommended (but a supplement that contains a blend of omega-3 and -6 may be necessary for therapeutic purposes). Canned fish, though still beneficial, contains lower levels of omega-3 than fresh. Shark, swordfish, king mackerel, and tilefish have also been found to contain significant amounts of mercury, and the U.S. Food and Drug Administration advises that young children should avoid eating these types of fish.

Fish is also a good source of choline – a nutrient needed (along with lecithin and B vitamins) to produce the brain chemical acetylcholine, vital for the rapid functioning of memory and improved learning ability. Shellfish is a good source of zinc, a crucial brain mineral for memory and concentration. Studies have shown that even a mild deficiency of zinc can impair mental function, leading to irritability, mood swings, and loss of appetite; when levels are replenished memory has been found to improve. Seafood also contains the amino acid tyrosine, which has been linked to increased mental energy and alertness, along with useful amounts of B vitamins, which are vital for energy production.

nutrient
KNOW-HOW

GOOD SOURCES OF COMPLEX CARBOHYDRATES

- Whole grain wheat
  - Brown rice
  - Wild rice
  - Millet
- Buckwheat
  - Quinoa
  - Barley
  - Oats
  - Rye

GRAINS & CEREALS

Children are particularly susceptible to the effects of fluctuating blood sugar levels; extreme highs and lows can lead to feelings of anxiety, light-headedness, irritability, poor concentration, and memory. Whole grains are the most nutritious option and, as complex carbohydrates, they are the body's main source of sustained energy. They also are good sources of all the key brain vitamins and minerals such as B vitamins, zinc, magnesium, folic acid, iron, selenium, and vitamin E. When refined as in white flour, pasta, and rice, grains and cereals lose many of their nutrients and also have an unsettling effect on blood sugar levels.

Complex carbohydrates help to boost levels of serotonin, the brain-calming, mood-enhancing chemical. A meal containing whole

Did you know?

PORTION SIZE

The World Health Organization now recommends that children eat five portions of fruit and vegetables a day – three portions of fruit and two of vegetables. But what is a portion of fruit or vegetables? Generally speaking, it is the amount a child can roughly fit into his or her hand. A glass of fresh fruit juice and a helping of beans both count as single portions.

wheat pasta, brown rice, noodles, or couscous may help children to wind down – ideal at the end of the day or if your child is very active or is a bad sleeper.

FRUITS & VEGETABLES

Fruits and vegetables provide an abundance of brain nutrients, particularly antioxidants and phytochemicals, a group of natural substances that have a range of therapeutic properties. Fruits and vegetables also contain a wide range of vitamins and minerals, and since increased vitamin and mineral intake has been found to improve IQ levels, particularly in children with a poor diet, it is vital to encourage your child to eat up his or her fruits and vegetables. Three portions of fruit and two of vegetables a day are recommended.

Fruit is a good source of vitamin C, boron, selenium, and carotenoids, while vegetables provide iron, vitamin C, calcium, selenium, B vitamins, magnesium, zinc, and boron.

Boron is responsible for producing positive brain waves, increasing alertness, and improving memory and concentration. Vitamin C aids the absorption of iron, which has been found to improve IQ and helps to energize the mind.

Many studies have shown that most children do not get enough fresh fruit and vegetables. It can be a struggle to get a child to "eat up his or her greens" – a struggle that most parents have experienced.

Easy ways to increase your child's consumption

One way around this problem is to offer your child a range of different fruits and vegetables. The greater choice he or she has, the more

chance there is of finding something your child really likes!

Try presenting fruits and vegetables in different ways. For example, children often will find sticks of raw vegetables more interesting and more palatable than cooked. Also, they can eat them with their hands rather than a boring knife and fork. Sticks also are good for dipping; serve them with a nutritious dip and you'll have twice the benefit.

If your children balk at the sight of certain vegetables, you can incorporate some, such as carrots, cabbage, sweet potato, peas, or even onion, into mashed potatoes. And if the going gets really tough, disguise puréed vegetables in sauces, soups, pies, or stews.

If the amount of fruits and vegetables you can get into your child is limited, then try to make sure it is as nutritious as possible. Buy the freshest you can – ideally organic, locally grown

Creating calm

The brain chemical serotonin has a mood-enhancing, calming effect and can induce sleepiness. Certain protein foods (turkey, chicken, eggs, lean meat, milk, cheese, and soybeans) contain the amino acid tryptophan, which is needed to produce serotonin. However, levels of serotonin depend upon how efficiently tryptophan is delivered to the brain. Peak levels of tryptophan may not reach the brain because other amino acids in the same foods compete against each other. However, carbohydrate foods (such as pasta or potatoes) eaten at the same time ease the path for the tryptophan to enter the brain cells and so raise serotonin levels.

This theory suggests that a meal based on carbohydrate foods accompanied by a moderate amount of protein can help to prepare the body for sleep. Conversely, a high-protein meal with a small amount of carbohydrate may have the opposite effect, keeping us alert. This is why a meal with a higher ratio of protein to carbohydrate is seen by some nutritionists as being better for breakfast and lunch, as it fuels the brain and stimulates the mind, while the ratio should be reversed for the evening meal. Other nutritionists, however, recommend that carbohydrate foods should always take pride of place on a plate.

produce – and make sure you don't keep it for too long before it's eaten. Steaming rather than boiling will help to preserve key brain nutrients.

NUTS & SEEDS

Just a handful of nuts and seeds can boost levels of B vitamins, iron, magnesium, calcium, vitamin E, selenium, potassium, zinc, and omega-6 essential fatty acids, important nutrients for brain function and energy production. Children who are lacking in the B vitamins may feel tired and lethargic and have trouble maintaining concentration. Nuts and seeds also are excellent sources of protein, but some varieties, such as peanuts, are high in saturated fat so should be eaten in moderation. Not only do nuts make a nutritious snack, but you also can use them to give a healthy boost to casseroles, stews, desserts, and cakes.

In Chinese medicine, walnuts are known as the "longevity fruit" and are an excellent brain food since they contain both omega-3 and omega-6 essential fatty acids (EFAs). Pumpkin seeds also include both types of EFA, while Brazil nuts, and sunflower and sesame seeds and their oils, are particularly rich in omega-6 fatty acids. Almonds, Brazil nuts, cashews, and hazelnuts are a good source of B vitamins. Buy unsalted nuts and those that are as fresh as you can find, preferably in their shells, since they can become rancid if stored for too long. Keep them fresh in an airtight container, away from the light.

OFF THE MENU

Nuts can be the cause of a severe allergy with life-threatening symptoms. If there is any history of nut allergy within your family, consult your doctor before giving nuts to your child. Children under five should not be given whole nuts due to the risk of choking.

BEANS, LEGUMES, & LENTILS

Excellent pantry essentials, beans, legumes, and lentils are often neglected at mealtimes – with the exception of baked beans, of course! If you find the prospect of all that overnight soaking off-putting, canned varieties make useful alternatives, but do choose those without added sugar and salt and make sure you rinse them before use.

Beans, legumes, and lentils are a valuable low-fat combination of protein and carbohydrates that also provide a good mix of mind- and memory-enhancing minerals, including B vitamins, calcium, iron, magnesium, manganese, and zinc. Tests have shown that children who eat adequate amounts of B vitamins will perform better in memory tests. Beans, legumes, and lentils are not classified as complete proteins, but including nuts and grains in the diet will ensure your child gets all the essential amino acids his or her body and mind need. Soybeans are an exception to the rule since, like meat and eggs, they are complete proteins. What's more, they also provide valuable omega-3 fats. Tofu, tempeh, and miso are all made from soybeans.

DAIRY FOODS

Cheese, milk, yogurt, and eggs are key protein foods, which are made up of essential amino acids, the building blocks of good health and mental vitality. Nevertheless, the saturated fat content of butter and cheese means that these should be eaten in moderation, since, in the long-term, they can clog the arteries that feed the brain. Dairy products are a good source of calcium and vitamins A and B. The brain-boosting amino acid tyrosine, which is converted into noradrenaline and dopamine, is found in milk and cheese and has been found to increase mental alertness and motivation. However, a milky drink at bedtime can be sleep-inducing, as the natural sugars in the milk (lactose) help to convert the tryptophan in the milk protein into the brain-calming substance serotonin. Children over two years of age can be given semiskim (1% or 2%) milk providing they are eating a well-balanced diet.

EGGS

Both nutritious and convenient, eggs provide lecithin, B vitamins, iron, and zinc, a powerful brain combo. You also can now buy eggs from hens whose feed has been fortified with omega-3 fatty acids, which could be useful if

Containing protein, carbohydrates, and several essential vitamins and minerals, beans, legumes, and lentils are tasty and versatile brain foods.

your offspring dislike fish. However, these do not come from free-range hens. Eggs are complete proteins, and so provide all the essential amino acids necessary to build neurotransmitters, the brain's messengers. They are also rich in tryptophan, needed to make the brain chemical serotonin, which calms the mind and acts as a sleep inducer.

MEAT & POULTRY

Animal proteins are classified as complete proteins, meaning that they contain all the eight essential amino acids. These are required to make key neurotransmitters in the brain believed to aid clarity of thought, concentration, and vitality. Red meat is an excellent source of iron, and studies have found that children are often deficient in this vital mineral, which can influence behavior and development. Increasing consumption of iron-rich foods has been found to lift mood, reduce anger, and improve IQ. Meat is also a good source of zinc, which along with iron helps to counteract the effect of lead in the body (a 1997 UK government report estimated that 10 percent of children have high enough blood lead levels to impair IQ). The downside is that red meat contains saturated fat, so cut off all visible fat and eat red meat only in moderate amounts.

Poultry is a low fat source of protein (as long as the skin is removed) and is also a good source of the amino acid tryptophan, important for the production of the brain-calming chemical serotonin. By eating a carbohydrate-based food at the same time, you will encourage the passage of tryptophan into the brain. Zinc is also found in chicken and turkey.

WATER

Most children don't drink enough fluids, especially while they are at school, but decent hydration is just as important for concentration, clarity of thought, and energy as a good balanced diet. A two percent loss in body fluids, for example, can cause a 20 percent reduction in both physical and mental performance. Choose from filtered or bottled water, diluted fresh fruit juice, or milk, and avoid carbonated sugary drinks. The amount of fluid a child needs depends on age and weight but, as a rough guide, the average 4- to 6-year-old should drink around five glasses a day and a 7- to 10-year-old should drink about six. A child who does not drink enough may experience headaches, lethargy, poor concentration, and constipation. Dehydration also affects the body's ability to transport essential nutrients throughout the body and brain.

Lethargy, headaches, poor concentration, and constipation are a few of the problems children can experience if their fluid intake is too low.

I can see a rainbow

The greater the variety of fruits and vegetables your child eats, the wider range of nutrients he or she will get. Make a game of choosing fruits and vegetables from the various color groups below and try to offer them in different guises: raw, steamed, or stir-fried, or in stews, sauces, or soups.

Tomatoes

RED

Tomatoes, strawberries, bell peppers, raspberries, apples, grapes, watermelon, cherries, radishes, rhubarb

ORANGE

Carrots, bell peppers, pumpkin, rutabaga, squash, sweet potato, oranges, tangerines, melon, nectarines, apricots

Pumpkin

YELLOW

Bananas, yellow zucchini, bell peppers, summer squash, bean sprouts, corn, pineapple, plums

Avocado

GREEN

Broccoli, brussels sprouts, cabbage, zucchini, avocado, apples, pears, salad leaves, spinach, peas, kiwi fruit

Bell peppers

PURPLE

Berries, eggplant, figs, plums, beets, red cabbage

Strawberries

Watermelon

Oranges

Peaches

Bananas

Grapes

Apples

Peas

Eggplant

Blueberries

Red cabbage

Brain DRAIN

Most parents are aware that diet plays an important role in their child's health. But it may come as a surprise to learn that a poor diet, lacking in nutrients, can be as bad for a child's mind as it is for his or her body. Without well-balanced and regular meals, the brain cannot work to its best ability and attention span, memory, and learning capabilities all suffer. A diet based on poor-quality burgers, chicken nuggets, French fries, potato chips, candy, cookies, and carbonated drinks will not provide children with the nutrients they need for healthy, active minds and bodies.

Did you know?

SUGAR ON LABELS

Sugar comes in various guises but it all has a similar effect on blood sugar levels. Sucrose, fructose, glucose, corn syrup, invert sugar, and dextrose are basically alternative names for refined sugar. Don't be tempted by labels promising "low-sugar" where manufacturers have replaced the sugar with artificial sweeteners such as aspartame or saccharin. These also have been linked with hyperactivity in children and can cause diarrhea.

SUGAR

One of the main culprits of "brain drain" is the refined sugar found in processed foods such as candy, cakes, cookies, and sweetened breakfast cereals. Refined sugar has little or no nutritional value and has even been found to "cloud" the brain when eaten in large quantities, not to mention the effect it has on tooth decay and weight gain. Highs and lows in blood sugar levels affect both mind and body. Eating a sugary food leads to a temporary surge in blood glucose levels, resulting in a rush of energy (think of kids after a birthday party) that is promptly followed by a slump or sugar-low (remember those tears and tantrums as they leave the party). It is this fluctuation that is said to produce an inconsistent supply of energy to the brain, leading to poor concentration and attention span, irritability, and fatigue.

Honey, molasses, and maple syrup are also forms of concentrated sugar, so have the same effect on blood sugar levels, although molasses is rich in certain minerals, and honey is believed to have some therapeutic properties.

Conversely, some researchers have found that sugar has a sedative effect. This may be because as a fast-releasing carbohydrate it stimulates the production of serotonin in the brain, making us feel drowsy a couple of hours after eating.

Sugary foods often include a fair amount of fat – just think of doughnuts, cookies, and chocolate bars. Fat takes a while to digest, so it can make brain function sluggish. In the long term, it also clogs the arteries, restricting blood flow to the brain.

Consuming large amounts of sugar also may inhibit the assimilation of certain nutrients, suppress the immune system, and lead to glucose intolerance, which means the body has problems regulating blood sugar levels. The symptoms include irritability, depression, crying spells, fatigue, poor concentration, and insomnia.

WHAT'S THE ALTERNATIVE?

Most children naturally will prefer sweet foods – to start with, breast milk is sweet – yet if eaten in moderation and as part of an overall well-balanced diet, this needn't be a problem. The main thing is to try and avoid over-processed sugary confections. Rather than cutting out sugar completely, which could lead to kids binging on candy whenever they get the opportunity, you can offer some healthier alternatives (see box, right). These will still influence blood sugar levels, but in most cases, these foods will also contain fiber and some protein to buffer the impact, as well as being good sources of vitamins and minerals.

JUNK FOODS

Admittedly, the definition of junk food is hazy, but it generally applies to highly processed, nutritionally deficient foods that are usually high in sugar, sweeteners, additives, or fat. It would be difficult, if not nigh on impossible, to remove all manufactured foods from our children's diets, but it is worth remembering that in the refining process many vitamins and minerals are destroyed that are vital for good brain health. Even when nutrients are artificially replaced, such as in breakfast cereals and breads, it is debatable whether they can be absorbed efficiently by the body.

Not only are most junk foods lacking in nutritional value, they are likely to contain artificial colors, preservatives, flavorings, salt, and sugar. They also tend to be high in saturated and hydrogenated fats, or "trans" fats. These slow down digestion, circulation, and mental processes, and clog the arteries, increasing the risk of diseases like heart disease and cancer.

• *Fresh or dried fruits. Snack-size portions of dried apricots, dates, or raisins are convenient for lunch boxes*

• *Small amounts of good-quality chocolate made with cocoa butter*

• *Oat bars, fruit cakes, crackers, or cookies made with whole grains*

• *Fresh fruit smoothies and milk shakes*

• *Fruit breads or English muffins made with whole wheat flour and topped with cream cheese*

• *Homemade popcorn*

• *Homemade or good-quality cakes*

• *Real-fruit or plain yogurt that you can flavor with homemade fruit purées or a spoonful of organic honey*

CAFFEINE

As well as being found in coffee and tea, caffeine is also found in chocolate – one bar can contain up to 50 mg – and some carbonated drinks, like cola. Caffeine is a stimulant and diuretic and can cause mood swings, since it affects the body's ability to

OFF THE MENU

- Mass-produced, poor-quality pizza, burgers, and sausages
- Processed cheese slices and "strings"
- Sliced meats with high-water, high-fat, and preservative content
- Breaded chicken or fish nuggets with low meat or fish content
- High-sugar breakfast cereals
- Highly flavored potato chips and reconstituted potato products
- Carbonated, sugary drinks such as cola and fruit-flavored drinks, or fruit drinks rather than fresh fruit juice
- Diet versions of drinks that contain artificial sweeteners
- Highly colored candies containing artificial colors and gelatin
- Poor-quality ice cream and highly colored ice popsicles
- Poor-quality artificially flavored yogurts
- High-sugar cereal bars or additive-laden, high-fat, and high-sugar cakes and cookies

CARBONATED DRINKS

Consumption of sweet, carbonated drinks is on the increase, yet there is nothing positive that can be said about most of them, with their added sugar, colors, sweeteners, caffeine, and preservatives. Carbonated drinks also are high in the mineral phosphorus, which inhibits calcium absorption. Calcium is vital for the production of the brain's messengers, neurotransmitters, which are said to have an effect on emotions.

ADDITIVES & PRESERVATIVES

A number of substances are routinely added to manufactured food to enhance taste, texture, and appearance, or to prolong shelf life. According to research, additives may adversely affect around one in seven children. Babies and young children are said to be especially vulnerable, since their systems are immature. While not all additives are potentially harmful, some of them have been linked to hyperactivity in sensitive children as well as being the potential cause of a range of allergies, poor memory, depression, and mood swings.

Avoiding additives altogether can be a minefield. Most potato chip manufacturers, for example, routinely add monosodium glutamate (MSG) to flavored varieties. This flavor enhancer has been linked to "Chinese restaurant syndrome," the symptoms of which are dizziness, anxiety, thirst, and mood swings.

The orange food coloring tartrazine (FD&C Yellow No. 5) is just one of the many additives known to influence behavior and possibly trigger the symptoms of ADHD (see page 30).

control blood sugar levels. One study carried out by researchers at the University of Bristol found that caffeine does not benefit mental performance in the long term. British school-children who were regularly given a cup of tea in the morning began to wake up feeling groggy and tired, were generally slower, and began to "need" a cup of tea in the morning – in the way that some adults do – to make their bodies and brains feel more alert and ready for the day.

Caffeine also depletes the body of certain B vitamins, zinc, potassium, calcium, and iron, all vital for good all-around cognitive performance.

Others include sunset yellow (FD&C Yellow No. 6), erythrosin (FD&C Red No. 3), benzoic acid, and sodium benzoate, as well as the previously mentioned MSG. The antioxidants BHA and BHT are also known to cause problems. A study carried out in Australia in 1994 found that 55 percent of children in their research who responded positively to the elimination of all food dyes and additives in their diet, reacted negatively when given a single dye again such as tartrazine. The children were more irritable, restless, and had sleep problems.

Many governments are dismissive of the case against additives, claiming that the evidence is contradictory and largely anecdotal, yet many parents who have cut out additives from their children's diets can counter this. Take, for example, the case of Michael and Christopher Parker, five-year-old identical twins. Michael was not allowed to eat snacks with dyes or preservatives for two weeks. He became noticeably calmer than his brother, who continued to follow his normal diet. Michael also appeared to show a 15-point increase in IQ over the period. When the study was extended to classmates, 57 percent of parents said that their children's behavior had shown an improvement.

Try to avoid foods containing additives, colors, and preservatives. If you are concerned that your child reacts adversely to food additives, keep a food diary and monitor his or her behavior over a period of time before contacting a doctor or dietitian.

THE ROLE OF ADDITIVES

ANTIOXIDANTS prevent food turning rancid.

COLORINGS add or intensify color (some are banned in the US).

EMULSIFIERS, STABILIZERS, THICKENERS, AND JELLING AGENTS affect the texture of food and bind ingredients together.

FLAVOR ENHANCERS enhance the flavor or smell of a food without adding any of their own.

PRESERVATIVES prevent and slow down deterioration in food. Any processed food with a long shelf life is likely to include preservatives.

HEAVY METALS AND PESTICIDES

Heavy metals such as lead, cadmium, mercury, and aluminum accumulate in the brain and have been linked to reduced intelligence, concentration, memory, and impulse control. Mercury dental fillings have also been linked to brain toxicity. Foods rich in zinc and selenium have been found to detoxify heavy metals in the body. See page 17 for good sources of these minerals.

The ultimate consequences of long-term exposure to pesticide residues is unknown but there is some evidence to suggest that in sensitive children pesticides may be linked to hyperactivity and allergies.

Food INTOLERANCES

One in ten children is thought to be affected by hyperactivity, also known as Attention Deficit Hyperactivity Disorder (ADHD), which may be aggravated by poor diet, while many children suffer intolerances or allergies to particular foods.

BEHAVIORAL PROBLEMS

The influence of diet on behavior is somewhat controversial, but poor diet, lack of essential fatty acids, and food allergies can certainly exacerbate symptoms, which may include destructive behavior, restlessness, poor concentration, learning difficulties, clumsiness, irritability, and poor social skills. For example, it

Essential nutrients

Research has found that children with ADHD are lacking in:

- *Essential fatty acids omega-3 and omega-6*

- *B-complex vitamins*

- *Chromium*

- *Zinc*

- *Magnesium*

- *Vitamin C*

has been suggested that children with ADHD often have problems with metabolizing sugar, the symptoms of which can be more pronounced in the morning when sugary foods are eaten on an empty stomach. When sugar is refined, it is also robbed of any mineral content, particularly chromium, which is needed to metabolize sugar and control blood glucose levels. This deficiency may cause bouts of hypoglycemia, leading to aggressive outbursts.

Deficiencies in zinc, calcium, and magnesium can cause restlessness, poor concentration, and learning difficulties, and a lack of these minerals also has been linked to children with ADHD.

Vitally important are the essential fatty acids omega-3 and -6. Numerous studies have shown that a deficiency in these fatty acids can lead to behavioral problems and learning difficulties and many children with ADHD have been found to have low levels of essential fatty acids. Research has found that boys are more likely to suffer from severe fatty-acid deficiency and have poorer reading and spelling abilities. Another study, still in its early stages, has linked depression and mood swings to omega-3 deficiency. Scientists suggest that these fatty acids may be able to suppress the signals that are responsible for sudden mood change. Increasing intake in the diet as well as through supplementation has been shown to improve brain metabolism and the symptoms of ADHD.

A lack of thiamine (vitamin B_1) is also linked to aggressive, erratic, and impulsive behavior. Potatoes, whole grains, nuts, seeds, eggs, meat, vegetables, and brown rice are good sources of B_1. Vitamin B_6 is equally important.

Numerous studies suggest there is a connection between food allergies or intolerances (see below) and behavioral problems, including ADHD. Some nutrition experts believe that sugar may not be the main factor when it comes to behavioral problems but that an allergy or intolerance to the additives, particularly colors, often used in sweets and sugary foods lies at the root of the problem. Eliminating food allergens has proved effective in treating children with ADHD.

ALLERGIES & INTOLERANCES

A food allergy occurs when the immune system overreacts to a normally harmless substance in a food by producing antibodies. It can cause a wide range of symptoms from a runny nose and diarrhea to a potentially life-threatening reaction such as swelling of the throat suffered by those who are allergic to nuts, for example. Somewhat confusingly, a child can test negatively for an allergy but may still react to certain foods. This is known as a food intolerance, which is often caused by a digestive problem.

Food intolerances are characterized by adverse reactions such as fuzzy-headedness, poor concentration, headaches, rashes, asthma,

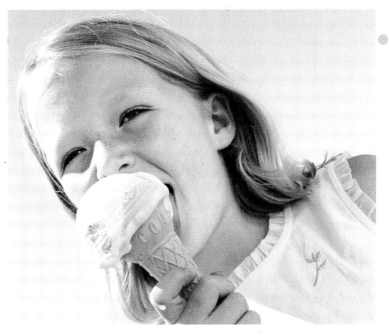

eczema, and behavioral problems that arise over hours or even days.

Allergies and intolerances tend to run in families, so if you or your partner suffers from an allergy or intolerance, then the chances are fairly likely that your child will develop one, too. Children are also more susceptible to food intolerances because of their immature digestive and immune systems. Reassuringly, while the number of cases of food intolerance appears to be increasing, the number of people with severe food allergies is still rare. The most common food allergens include dairy products, eggs, tomatoes, citrus fruit, wheat, nuts, soy, and shellfish. Always consult your doctor or dietitian about allergy testing and before eliminating any food from your children's diets.

Dairy products are one of the most common causes of food allergies, but there are several nondairy substitutes available.

Best BUYS

So far, this book has concentrated on the individual nutrients and foods that can benefit your child and the substances that will hold back his or her progress. Now it's time to consider how you shop for food. Buy it wisely and your children will get the maximum nutritional benefits from their food.

Farmers markets are popular and provide a great way of ensuring you buy the freshest, best-quality, locally grown produce.

Concerns about chemicals in our food mean that many of us are opting for organic produce. Since it's believed that children are more vulnerable to the effects of pesticide residues than adults (see box, page 29), buying organic food for them makes even more sense. You may have to pay slightly more for organic products, but they are generally tastier, fresher, and more nutritious.

FRUITS & VEGETABLES

Whenever you shop for fruits and vegetables, you need to buy the freshest you can get. The longer fruits and vegetables are left hanging around, the less nutrients they will contain. Therefore, it's a good idea to shop in stores that have a high turnover. Try to avoid fruits and vegetables that have been displayed outdoors or in a hot, lighted window, since nutrient levels will have diminished. Fluorescent lighting can have the same effect.

Most supermarkets sell a good selection of organic fruits and vegetables. Organic fruits and vegetables tend to taste better because they are not intensively grown and so do not absorb excessive water. Some studies have shown that the lower levels of water in organic fruits and vegetables means that they contain a higher concentration of vitamins and minerals. Organic produce is generally grown in better quality soil and left to ripen longer on the plant, rather than being artificially ripened, which can affect flavor and nutrient levels.

There was a time when organic produce was difficult to find in stores because organic farmers were few and far between. Fortunately, some supermarkets are beginning to stock more and more locally grown produce. For

IS IT FRESH?

Some fruits and vegetables are older than they look! Apples can be stored for up to 12 months in a controlled-temperature atmosphere. Likewise, carrots can be around for up to nine months, while potatoes can be up to 12 months old if kept in cold storage. Potatoes intended for long-term storage may also be sprayed with a chemical sprout inhibitor. Apples and oranges are also routinely waxed to give them a sheen and seal in moisture, after which they are hot-air dried. Look for organic, seasonal, and preferably local fruit and vegetables. Buy unwaxed fruit if possible. Look for firm, unblemished produce and be slightly suspicious of special offers, since they may indicate that the retailer has a surplus of produce near its sell-by date.

fresh local food, you could also try farmers markets, food co-ops, or buying direct from the farms themselves – this is also often a cheaper way to buy organic.

Wherever you shop, it's a good idea to buy fruits and vegetables in small quantities on a regular basis. Choose loose produce, as it will be much easier to check for quality – and you won't be taking home unwanted packaging. Remember to remove the goods from any plastic bags when storing.

MEAT, FISH, & EGGS

Worries about what's been put in meat or fish and where it's come from mean that many families are already choosing organic options. Organic meat and poultry comes from animals that are not routinely fed antibiotics and hormones, and that have been farmed under higher standards of animal welfare and with strict controls on feed. No genetically engineered ingredients are allowed. Because meat is high in saturated fat, purchase leaner cuts such as fillet of beef.

Sausages make a quick, convenient lunch or supper, but they do vary hugely in quality. Buy the most expensive products you can afford with the highest quantity of meat, preferably organic, and with few fillers and additives. The same goes for bacon and the like. There are vegetarian alternatives available, but these can contain an alarming number of unwanted additives.

When buying fish, wild or organically farmed fish are preferable to those farmed conventionally, which may have been given pesticides and additives such as colors – just look at the difference in color between farmed and wild salmon. Undyed smoked haddock and smoked cod are also better choices than their bright yellow alternatives.

When shopping for fresh fish and meat, it is easier to check quality and freshness if you buy over the counter – whether it's in the supermarket, butcher, or at a farmers market.

When buying eggs, look for organic and free-range, which will come from hens kept in preferable living conditions that are given a natural diet and not routinely fed on antibiotics or yolk-enhancing dyes. Cartons depicting attractive countryside scenes or including the words "farm fresh" mean little – the eggs are just as likely to come from battery farms. Store eggs in the refrigerator, where they will keep for a couple of weeks.

PACKAGED OR PREPARED FOODS

If you're buying packaged or prepared foods you need to check the labeling to see what ingredients and additives they contain. You want to avoid those with high amounts of sugar, saturated and hydrogenated (trans) fats, artificial colors and flavoring, additives, preservatives, and artificial sweeteners, many of which have been linked to behavioral problems, hyperactivity, and food allergies in children.

Fish fingers, chicken nuggets, and burgers are popular with children but are highly processed and likely to contain substantial amounts of fat, salt, artificial colors, and additives. There are no official rules covering such products, which means that they don't have to include a specified percentage of meat

(often they contain less than 40 percent) and they tend to be made with chopped, re-formed, or shaped meat.

Choose fish without batter or bread crumbs, which can be an excuse for manufacturers to add colors, preservatives, fat, and cheap fillers, or if you can't resist the crumbed version, look for the brand with the highest fish content and lowest number of additives and artificial colors (or make your own homemade bread crumbs). Bear in mind that when you look at the list on a label, the first ingredient is the one found in the highest quantity.

Pizzas are perfect ready-made meals – take them straight from the refrigerator or freezer and they cook in a matter of minutes – but they are often seen as junk food. Of course, many of the pizzas on sale are, but it is increasingly easy to find decent-quality pizzas made with natural ingredients. Delis often sell delicious homemade pizza by the slice, and of course you can make your own; see page 61.

PANTRY, REFRIGERATOR, AND FREEZER FOODS

When you've got hungry mouths to feed, you don't want to be popping out to the store before every meal, so make sure your cupboards, refrigerator, and freezer are kept well stocked. Below we set out the best stand-bys to have on hand so you can plan meals that are healthy and nutritious for your children.

Cereal staples

Pasta must be one of the ultimate convenience foods – easy to cook and the perfect base for so many meals. It's also very popular with most children. There is a huge range of different shapes to try, as well as colored pasta – just make sure you buy the sort with natural coloring (such as spinach and tomato). Dried pasta keeps well stored in an airtight container and you can keep fresh pasta in the freezer.

Rice and noodles also are ideal starting points for many dishes and you might find it useful to have more than one kind of rice in stock. Keep a long-grain or easy-cook rice (preferably brown) to make pilafs or to serve with curries and stir-fries, some arborio or carnaroli rice for making risotto, and a short-grain rice for some good old-fashioned rice puddings. And don't forget couscous and buckwheat – so easy to cook and turn into delicious meals with just a few flavorings. Add a spoonful of pesto, some chopped herbs, or

some raisins and toasted nuts. Or make a warm salad of grains by stirring in some chopped tomato, cucumber, and feta cheese.

Breakfast cereals are a vital item in any family's pantry. They're a convenient way to give your children a healthy start in the morning – if you choose wisely. Avoid sugar-rich cereals and opt for sugar-free or low-sugar, whole-grain cereals.

Canned and packaged foods

Some canned vegetables can be a useful alternative to fresh or frozen vegetables. Children often love corn, and the canned type is convenient and readily available. Look for the no-added-sugar and no-added-salt versions and rinse well before using. Canned lentils and beans, already soaked and cooked, cut down cooking time by hours.

Baked beans are a popular quick meal for children and adults alike, so a few cans of organic baked beans are a useful standby. Look for brands that are lower in salt and sugar, but try to avoid artificial sweeteners added in place of sugar. Half a small can of baked beans counts as one of the recommended five daily portions of fruits and vegetables.

A variety of fish comes canned, such as sardines, mackerel, salmon, and tuna, all of which can be turned into tasty meals or sandwich fillings. They're also a good source of those omega-3 fatty acids, albeit in lower amounts than found in fresh fish.

Canned soup can be high in salt and sugar and it's relatively quick to make your own. If you use bouillon cubes or powder, avoid those that are high in salt and contain artificial colors and sugar, and made with wholly organic ingredients.

High-fruit, no-added-sugar jams and spreads have an intensively fruity flavor and a higher ratio of fruit to sugar than cheaper alternatives. They may be slightly more expensive but they are worth it in terms of fruit content and flavor. You will need to keep them in the refrigerator, as they won't keep in the same way as traditional jams.

Nut butters such as peanut, cashew, or hazelnut provide an energy-dense snack if spread on bread or English muffins. Look for those brands that have the fewest additives and no added sugar. Unsalted nuts and seeds also make convenient snacks, but don't give children under five whole nuts, and avoid them altogether if there is any history of nut allergy in your family. Try toasting nuts and seeds to add to their flavor. Nuts quickly become rancid once shelled, so buy them in the shells and store them in an airtight container until needed.

Dried fruit is an energy-packed source of vitamins and minerals, including iron. The choice is extensive but look for unsulfured fruit. Sulfur dioxide is used as a preservative and can provoke asthma attacks in susceptible children. Dried fruit is a valuable ingredient in many dishes, both sweet and savory, and small packs of dried fruit are perfect for lunch boxes or snacks.

Bread sticks, rice, oat or corn cakes make ideal snacks and are healthier alternatives to salty and fatty potato chips and

and flavoring. Keep a few packages of miso soup in the cupboard. Just add hot water to the powdered miso and then pour over noodles and steamed vegetables. Sprinkle with some sesame seeds for a quick, healthy meal.

Treats and snacks

You can't keep kids away from some of those little treats that make mealtimes more fun for them. You can, however, find healthier versions of some of their favorites. Tomato ketchup, for example, now comes in many different forms and you can get a very tasty version that's lower in both salt similar snacks. Try to avoid those that contain artificial additives such as the flavor enhancer monosodium glutamate – the fewer the ingredients the better.

You also can buy a range of fruit bars, low-sugar cereal bars, or natural fruit leathers that are useful to keep for snacks and lunch boxes. These are preferable to the high-sugar, high-color, high-additive, gelatin-filled alternatives generally available.

And last but not least, keep everyone happy with some good-quality chocolate. A popular treat with all the family as well as a vital cooking ingredient, bittersweet chocolate contains at least 50 percent cocoa solids and milk chocolate contains between 15 and 30 percent. Avoid bars with unwanted additives, and if buying white chocolate, choose bars made with pure cocoa butter, not vegetable fat.

REFRIGERATED FOODS

When you're rustling up a meal – whether it's a quick supper or a Sunday dinner – the refrigerator is usually your first port of call. Where would we be without eggs, milk, and cheese – all of which keep best when chilled? Eggs are ideal for a light meal as well as being an essential ingredient in many recipes. Butter and nonhydrogenated spreads are preferable to margarines and spreads containing trans, or hydrogenated, fats and other additives, which are just as bad for our health as saturated fat.

Cheese is a perfect standby ingredient – use it to top pizzas or make macaroni and cheese, or keep some for snacks. Avoid heavily processed cheeses, so often aimed at children, and buy good-quality, preferably organic, cheese.

Small-size portions of items like ham and cheese, aimed at children's lunch boxes, are easy to find. However, these are usually high in artificial additives and are best avoided. Instead, buy good-quality ham, pâté, or cheese when you want something to pop in your child's lunch box.

A tub of hummus is a great snack and lunch standby. Give it to children with strips of pita bread or carrot sticks for a healthy dip, or put it in their sandwiches. You even can stir it into soups and stews for added flavor. Use pesto in the same way or stir it into pasta, rice, or even mashed potatoes for a real change.

It's always a good idea to have some yogurt in the refrigerator for a quick and easy dessert. However, some brands contain little fruit and are often laden with added color, flavor, sugar, artificial sweeteners, and gelatin. Go for those

ACTIVE-CULTURE YOGURTS

Most of us are familiar with the active-culture yogurts now available, but why do we need them? A healthy intestine is very important and ensures that foods are digested well and nutrients are transported to where they are needed. The healthy bacteria in active-culture yogurts may help the immune system to resist gastric bugs and, if eaten after a course of antibiotics, may restore the internal flora of the intestine – which is particularly important for children.

that contain real fruit. If you keep a large pot of plain yogurt in the refrigerator you can flavor it yourself. Try chopped banana, homemade fresh fruit purées, toasted nuts and seeds, or a spoonful of maple syrup.

Tofu (also known as soybean curd) is a useful standby, especially if anyone in your family is a vegetarian. Rich in calcium and a good source of protein, it can be very versatile. Try it roasted or stir-fried, after marinating in black bean sauce or a mixture of garlic, ginger, honey, and sesame oil.

Soup makes a wonderful quick meal, but canned and packaged soups are best avoided, since they tend to be high in sugar and salt. If you want to buy ready-made soup, go for the "fresh" soups from the refrigerated section and store them in the refrigerator or freezer.

Frozen vegetables can contain higher amounts of nutrients, such as vitamin C and iron than fresh produce since they are often

frozen very soon after picking, whereas fresh vegetables may be around for quite a while before they land on our plates. Therefore, a few packs of frozen vegetables make a valuable addition to any freezer. Broccoli, lima beans, spinach, corn, or carrots are all useful standbys, as are, of course, peas – sometimes the only vegetable that some kids will eat!

DRINKS

There are now so many different types of fruit juice around that choosing the most natural and healthiest can be tricky. The best way to get beneficial amounts of vitamins without additives is to make fruit juice at home from good-quality, organic fresh fruit. If you have a juicer and a freezer, you can make some in batches and freeze to store.

In supermarkets you'll find chilled, freshly squeezed juices or smoothies and these contain useful amounts of vitamins, although some are destroyed in the manufacturing process. Be aware that bottles and cartons labeled as fruit drinks can contain as little as five percent fruit juice, along with added sugar or artificial sweeteners and additives. Remarkably, some fruit-flavored drinks contain no real fruit at all. They may have added vitamins but this does not make them healthy drinks. And watch out for those drinks sold in the refrigerated section that are masquerading as real fruit juice – they're not all that they seem!

Bear in mind that all fruit juices and drinks contain sugar, whether it is natural or not, so can cause tooth decay. Dilute juice with water or only serve at mealtimes and get children to brush their teeth regularly.

Cooking SMART

The way you cook and prepare food influences its nutritional content. Certain cooking methods will preserve nutrients, cut out excess fat, and protect against disease-causing organisms. Make sure any frozen products are thoroughly defrosted before cooking.

VEGETABLES

Generally speaking, eating raw fruit and vegetables will be most beneficial. Make sure you wash vegetables before using, but do not soak them because water-soluble nutrients will leach into the water. Hold root vegetables such as carrots under cold running water and use a vegetable scrubbing brush to clean thoroughly. Many nutrients are found in or just below the skin, so avoid peeling them, if at all possible. If your children like their vegetables peeled, you can cook them in their skins first and then peel them.

When you're making a meal, it's best not to prepare vegetables too far in advance of cooking or serving, as nutrients, such as vitamin C, will diminish as soon as the cut surface is exposed to air. The same is true of fruit. Once cooked, serve vegetables as soon as possible because they will begin to lose their nutritional content if they stand.

Steaming or stir-frying is preferable to boiling – the latter destroys water-soluble vitamins such as B and C. Cooking vegetables whole or in large pieces helps to preserve their nutritional content. Keep the cooking water and use it as a stock.

MEAT

As well as choosing leaner cuts, you also should trim off all extra visible fat. This will reduce the cooking time by about 20 percent. Fat-free cooking methods such as stewing, braising, or broiling are best. If you are making a casserole, you should skim off the fat at regular intervals. If you are going to fry meat, which is best avoided, make sure you use olive or canola oil in place of butter. Both these oils are high in monounsaturated fats. Alternatively, use a non-stick frying pan. Place roasting meats on a rack to allow fat to drip off while cooking.

POULTRY

Rinse the poultry thoroughly, including the cavity if you are cooking a whole bird. If roasting a whole bird, prick the skin to allow the fat to run out, and place on a rack. Make sure poultry is cooked thoroughly to protect against any possibility of salmonella poisoning. If using a thermometer, it should read 180°F for a whole bird (in the thickest part) and 170°F for pieces. Alternatively, pierce the poultry with a fork and make sure the juices run clear. Stir-frying, poaching, and baking are low-fat cooking methods. Always remove the skin before serving, as this contains high levels of fat.

*Meal*TIMES

For mental clarity, sustained energy levels, and concentration, it's not just what children eat that matters but when. Children are particularly vulnerable to dips in blood sugar levels, which can lead to mood swings, irritability, and poor attention. Regular healthy meals, supplemented by nutritious snacks and sufficient fluids, are crucial throughout the day to maintain steady blood sugar levels.

BREAKFAST

It is now widely recognized by nutrition experts, and supported by research, that children who eat a decent breakfast perform better at school. Breakfast is seen as the most important meal of the day, since it replenishes vital brain nutrients and blood sugar (glucose) levels that are depleted overnight. Breakfast also kick-starts the metabolism, which slows down overnight. Moreover, research has shown that skipping the first meal of the day can lead to children developing an unhealthy pattern of snacking on high-fat, high-sugar foods. This is particularly true of children who leave the house on empty

Breakfast ideas

Nutritionists say that the perfect breakfast should satisfy the appetite and provide long-term energy without being too high in fat or giving an immediate sugar rush – which is what would happen if you gave children a sugar-laden breakfast cereal. It should provide 25 percent of a child's daily nutrient requirement. Turn to page 49 for breakfast recipes, but other quick suggestions to start the day include:

- *Oatmeal with sliced banana*

- *Boiled or poached egg on wholewheat toast*

- *Low-sugar breakfast cereal with fruit and milk*

- *Fresh fruit smoothie*

- *Yogurt with fruit*

- *Beans on wholewheat toast*

- *Broiled tomato and bacon or sausages with wholewheat toast*

- *Pancakes made with wholewheat flour, topped with fruit*

- *Whole wheat English muffin or bread with low-sugar jam or peanut butter*

- *Poached or grilled fish*

stomachs and stop to buy candy and other snacks on the way to school.

Many studies show that, compared to children who do eat breakfast, those who skip this meal do not perform as well in areas such as numeracy, problem solving, information selection and recall, and language skills. This is because the body needs fuel on waking, and when it doesn't get the sustenance it needs, it switches to survival mode and releases energy only for emergencies. This means that the body and, more specifically, the brain are without the glucose they so badly need. Symptoms such as lack of concentration and poor memory are indications that the brain is struggling due to low levels of fuel.

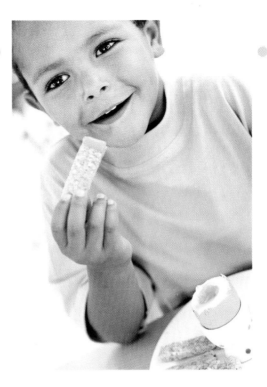

CARBOHYDRATES OR PROTEIN?

In the main, it is believed that the positive influence of breakfast on brain function is because the meal is usually based on carbohydrates – breakfast cereals and toast are good examples. Cereals are often fortified with vitamins and minerals, including the B vitamins and iron, which help with energy production. They also provide glucose, which is the main fuel for the brain, while the milk poured over cereal is a good source of calcium, B-complex vitamins, zinc, and magnesium.

Controversially, there is also research to suggest that a protein-based breakfast is more successful in stimulating the brain and satisfies the appetite quicker and for longer than a carbohydrate meal. It's believed that this is because the protein meal encourages the release of chemicals that increase alertness and boost reaction times. This means that protein foods such as eggs, milk, yogurt, beans, and fish may play a greater role in getting the brain fired up in the morning. The best policy, since the ratio of protein to carbohydrate is unknown, is to make sure you include both in each meal, and that includes breakfast.

LUNCH

A wholesome lunch, whether it be home-cooked, packed, or a school lunch, is vital for maintaining energy levels and sustaining memory, concentration, and learning for the

nutrient
KNOW-HOW

QUICK SNACK IDEAS

- Whole wheat English muffin with mashed banana
- Whole grain crackers with cream cheese
- French toast
- Boiled egg with toast fingers
- Peanut butter on sesame-seed bagel
- Hummus and vegetable sticks
- Dried fruit and nuts
- Roasted sunflower and pumpkin seeds
- Fruit sticks: slices of apple, melon, peach
- Handful of grapes or strawberries

rest of the day. School meals have been the target of criticism for some time, and many local authorities have addressed these concerns by ensuring there are healthy options among the French fries, fish sticks, and beans. Unfortunately, where children are able to select their own lunches, these healthier alternatives are often ignored. What's more, children are usually unfamiliar with the rules of a balanced diet and tend to overload their plates with the highly refined carbohydrate, high-fat options.

If you're able to send your child to school with a packed lunch, this is often a good way of monitoring his or her diet. When time is short, it can be tricky to be inspired about packed lunches and it's very easy to get stuck in the "sandwich, potato chips, chocolate bar, and an apple" rut. Variety is the key; try offering different types of fruit, half an avocado, a kiwifruit, cubes of melon, or dried fruit, for example. There are plenty of different kinds of bread to choose from such as tortillas, mini rolls, bagels, ciabatta, or English muffins. A thermos is perfect for holding soup for a warming winter lunch or try rice, potato, or pasta salads. See pages 44–5 for more tips and ideas for lunch boxes.

Following on from the controversial research that suggests breakfast should include a higher ratio of protein to carbohydrate, some nutritionists believe that lunch should adopt similar guidelines. Proteins are believed to be better for mental stimulation and alertness and will help to avoid the mid-afternoon dip in energy that many children experience. On the other hand, the general rule is that carbohydrates, which are converted into glucose, are the brain's most important source of fuel and should play a major part in every meal throughout the day.

SNACKS

In the past, dietitians have discouraged eating between meals, but there is mounting evidence to suggest that kids need to eat little and often, since stores of glucose are used up more quickly in children than in adults. In fact it's good for children to have a couple of snacks – albeit healthy ones – during the day to maintain brain efficiency by keeping blood sugar levels steady. Avoid the short-term boost given by high-fat, high-sugar snacks and drinks. The sugar high is followed by a sugar slump, often resulting in mood swings and irritability. It also may be beneficial to provide a carbohydrate-based snack such as toast or an English muffin an hour or two before bedtime, since carbohydrates are said to encourage the production of the calming brain chemical serotonin. A snack will also keep hunger at bay during the night, since dips in blood sugar levels may be one reason for a child waking in the night.

DINNER

Originating from the same study that suggested we should eat more protein at breakfast and lunch is the finding that dinner should include a higher proportion of carbohydrate to protein. Carbohydrates, such as pasta, rice, couscous, and potatoes, trigger the release of the brain chemical serotonin, which is said to induce feelings of calm and encourage sleep (see page 23). If your child is particularly active or hyper at the end of the day, it could be well worth increasing the amount of carbohydrates he or she eats at this time. However, don't forget the importance of protein, too. It's vital to eat a variety of protein-rich foods to get a balance of the essential amino acids that have to be provided by diet and are necessary for building the brain's messengers. Opt for good-quality organic meat, fish, eggs, beans, lentils, cheese, nuts, and seeds. For many children, this is the main meal of the day, and it can be an opportunity to encourage your child to top up his or her intake of fruit and vegetables to reach the recommended daily intake of five portions.

LUNCH BOXES

Though many parents dread the daily grind of coming up with something edible to put into the lunch box, with a little advance planning, a packed lunch can make a major contribution to a well-rounded healthy diet.

THE TRIMMINGS

It may sound odd to pay attention to the box itself, before discussing what goes in it, but appearances are more important to children than most adults care to acknowledge. You are more likely to receive a favorable uptake on your packed lunch if you provide an attractive container and appropriate cutlery and napkin, where necessary. Choose a rigid lunch box to protect the contents and only buy a box with a decorative theme if it is age appropriate and if your child approves. Some boxes contain freezer aids to help keep food cool, which is a good idea, especially in summer. Boxes also come divided into compartments, which seems a useful idea until you try to force food into each slot. A thermos can be useful for keeping soups warm and drinks cool depending on the season.

AVERAGE CHOICE

It's incredibly easy to be misled by food industry claims when short on time and inspiration. The following food products may have promised much but deliver little.

- Concentrated fruit drinks corrode tooth enamel and are low in fruit content.

- Bananas are a perfect source of energy but are lunch box nightmares – if they aren't squashed they turn black and ooze over other food.

- Many manufactured cereal bars contain little "slow-release" energy. They are high in sugar and calories and are expensive.

- White bread has had fiber and nutrients removed. Its filling, "processed meat," is heavy on additives to provide flavor and contains the cheapest cuts of meat.

- Cartons of fruit dessert contain little fruit, lots of refined sugar, and are not filling.

- Potato chips are high in fat and many additives. If you opt for low fat, be aware that it is usually replaced by sugar or chemical binding agents.

BEST CHOICE

The contents of the lunch box below reflect how you should think about nutritional content. You need to include both protein and carbohydrates to provide energy throughout the day and to aid concentration, memory, IQ, and attention span. Fresh fruits and vegetables are also a must.

Vary the contents as much as possible, and if you know your child dislikes a food, resist the temptation to keep slipping it in in the hope he will eat it, however good it may be for him.

● Diluted fresh fruit juice or water are preferable to concentrates or carbonated drinks in terms of tooth decay and calories; energy should always be provided by slow-release foods rather than liquids. Good hydration is essential to maintain concentration.

● Yogurt in a tube acts as a cooler stick if prefrozen. Only buy those with a high real fruit content. Alternatively, make your own flavored variety – stir a fruit purée or coulis into a pot of yogurt with live and active cultures.

● Vitamin C-rich fruit will encourage iron absorption and aid energy production.

● Celery and carrot sticks as well as red pepper, cucumber, snow peas, etc., provide a range of vitamins and can be dipped into yogurt dips or hummus.

● By making your own cereal bars (see page 50) you can control the ingredients used and save money.

● Stone-ground whole wheat bread provides extra roughage and is more nutritious than white. Butter can quickly become "sweaty," so try a thin spread of mayonnaise to provide a creamy taste or add extra lettuce to prevent fillings from tasting dry. Cheese, egg, canned fish, turkey, or good-quality ham are healthy options and provide a protein boost.

Brainboosting
RECIPES

These recipes are created with children in mind, but will also be enjoyed by adults, which will make all family meals easier to prepare and more fun to enjoy. They contain the foods that are said to be most beneficial for the brain and those that have been shown, in some instances, to improve IQ, memory, attention span, and concentration.

A GOOD START

The most important meal of the day, breakfast replenishes vital brain nutrients and energy depleted overnight. Recent research suggests that children who eat a decent breakfast perform better at school.

FRUIT & NUT CLEVER CLUSTERS

Most breakfast cereals contain excessive amounts of sugar and, perhaps surprisingly, salt – a bowl of cornflakes can contain more sodium than a bag of potato chips! Try making this crunchy cereal – it's a type of granola that's a nutritious mixture of fruits, nuts, oats, and seeds, providing plenty of sustained energy for the day ahead. You can easily adapt this recipe to include favorite dried fruits.

About 20 portions
¾ cup whole hazelnuts
½ cup blanched almonds
3 cups oats
½ cup sunflower seeds
¼ cup sesame seeds
3 tbsp omega-blend oil or sunflower oil
6 tbsp honey
¾ cup chopped dried dates
¾ cup ready-to-eat unsulfured dried
  apricots, roughly chopped
milk or yogurt with live and active
  cultures, to serve

1 Preheat the oven to 275°F. Place the hazelnuts and almonds in a plastic bag and crush with a rolling pin until roughly broken. Place the crushed nuts in a bowl with the oats and seeds.
2 Heat the oil and honey gently in a saucepan until the honey has just melted. Stir the mixture into the oats, nuts, and seeds.

BRAIN BOX

Nuts and seeds contain plenty of brainboosting nutrients, being an excellent source of B-complex vitamins, iron, vitamin E, zinc, selenium, and omega-6 essential fatty acids. **Whole oats** are a complex carbohydrate that help to keep blood sugar levels steady, enabling the brain to work more efficiently.

3 Spread the mixture in an even layer on two baking sheets and bake for 35 minutes, stirring occasionally, until golden and slightly crisp (the mixture will become crispier as it cools).
4 Transfer the mixture to a bowl and mix in the dates and apricots, then leave to cool. Store in an airtight container until ready to eat. Serve with milk or yogurt.

WONDER CRUNCH

A muesli-type cereal featuring a brain-nurturing combination of whole grains, nuts, seeds, and fruit, hence the name.

About 20 portions
¾ cup slivered almonds
½ cup Brazil nuts, chopped
½ cup sunflower seeds
scant ½ cup pumpkin seeds
1 14-oz box wheat flakes
1½ cups unsulfured dried apricots,
  finely chopped
1¼ cups raisins

1 Lightly toast the almonds, Brazil nuts, sunflower seeds, and pumpkin seeds in a dry frying pan over medium heat for 3 minutes, stirring frequently, until golden. Leave to cool.
2 Combine the toasted nuts and seeds, wheat flakes, and dried fruit in a large bowl; mix well. Transfer to a baking sheet to cool, and store in an airtight container. Serve with milk, or yogurt with live and active cultures, and fresh fruit.

BRAIN BOX

Wheat flakes provide a rich array of nutrients and although mainly a complex carbohydrate food, they also contain a certain amount of protein, both of which are essential fuel for the brain and keep energy and blood sugar levels steady.

POWER BREAKFAST BARS

Breakfast is undoubtedly the most important meal of the day, replenishing the brain after a night's sleep. Yet when time is short – especially on school days – this oat, apple, and seed cereal bar can be a real boon. Serve with a glass of milk or fresh fruit juice.

Makes 10 bars

1 stick unsalted butter
generous ½ cup light brown sugar
4 tbsp golden syrup or honey
2½ cups rolled oats
2 tbsp sunflower seeds
1 tbsp sesame seeds
1 tbsp pumpkin seeds
1 eating apple, pared, cored, and grated

1 Preheat the oven to 350°F. Grease and line an 8-in-square cake pan. Melt the butter in a saucepan over a low heat and add the sugar and syrup or honey. Heat until just warm – do not allow to boil.
2 Put the oats, seeds, and apple in a mixing bowl and pour on the buttery syrup. Mix well until combined and spoon the mixture into the prepared pan.
3 Bake for 25–30 minutes until golden and slightly crisp. Cut into 10 bars while still warm and leave in the pan until cool and crisp.

BANANA YOGURT

This simple breakfast provides plenty of brain-sustaining protein as well as essential vitamins and minerals for the day ahead. Yogurt with live and active cultures contains beneficial bacteria that restores equilibrium to the digestive system, especially following a course of antibiotics or a stomach upset. It also helps to increase the uptake of nutrients.

Serves 2

2 tbsp mixed seeds such as sunflower, pumpkin, and sesame
2 small ripe bananas
1 cup yogurt with live and active cultures
2 tsp maple syrup

1 Lightly toast the seeds in a dry frying pan until just golden, tossing frequently.
2 Slice the bananas into two glasses or bowls. Top with the yogurt, then sprinkle with the seeds. Drizzle each serving with the maple syrup.

BRAIN BOX

Despite their size, **seeds** are a powerhouse of brain nutrients, particularly omega-6 essential fatty acids (pumpkin seeds also provide omega-3), zinc, magnesium, and vitamin E.

APPLE CROISSANT

The lightly spiced apple compote makes a delicious filling for a croissant. It can also be puréed and stirred into yogurt with live and active cultures for a healthy change from store-bought yogurts.

Serves 2
2 eating apples, pared, cored, and
   roughly diced
½ tsp ground cinnamon
small pat of butter
squeeze fresh lemon juice
6 tbsp water
2 croissants
sprinkling of toasted almonds
yogurt with live and active cultures,
   to serve

1 Put the apples, cinnamon, butter, lemon juice (this prevents the apple browning), and water in a heavy-based, nonmetallic saucepan. Simmer, half-covered, over medium heat for 20 minutes, until the apples are tender. Lightly mash the apples with a fork to break them down slightly.
2 Warm the croissants, split in half, and spoon the apples on top. Sprinkle with toasted almonds and serve with a spoonful of yogurt.

VERY MERRY BERRY YOGURT

Many children dislike "bits" in their food, which unfortunately can put them off berries. This compote is sieved to remove any offending seeds and skin, resulting in an intensely fruity red sauce. It is delicious stirred into a yogurt with live and active cultures, with a sprinkling of granola.

Serves 2–4
2 cups mixed berries such as
   strawberries or raspberries
1–2 tbsp superfine sugar, to taste
1 tbsp cornstarch
Fruit & Nut Clever Clusters (see page
   49), to serve
yogurt with live and active cultures,
   to serve

1 Rinse then hull the fruit. Purée the mixed berries in a food processor or

blender. Sieve the purée into a pan to remove any skin and seeds. Add a little sugar and the cornstarch to the pan and heat gently and briefly, stirring frequently, until thickened. Taste and add a little more sugar, if necessary.
2 Place a few spoonfuls of the Fruit & Nut Clever Clusters in a glass or bowl, top with a few spoonfuls of yogurt, then some berry purée. Top with more yogurt and a final sprinkling of Fruit & Nut Clusters.

OATMEAL WITH APRICOT SAUCE

A bowl of warming oatmeal makes a perfect start to the day. Oats are digested slowly in the body, helping to maintain energy levels by keeping blood sugar levels steady. Sprinkle with a few linseeds before serving, if desired.

Serves 2
1 cup rolled oats
1 tsp wheat germ (optional)
1½ cups milk
2 tsp clear honey, to serve (optional)
a sprinkling of linseeds (or flaxseeds), to serve (optional)

for the apricot sauce:
1 cup ready-to-eat unsulfured apricots, roughly chopped
⅔ cup fresh apple juice
⅔ cup water

1 To make the apricot sauce, place the apricots in a saucepan with the apple juice and water. Bring to a boil, cover, then reduce the heat and simmer for 30 minutes or until the apricots are tender. Place the apricots and any liquid left in the pan in a blender or food processor and purée until smooth. Set aside to cool.
2 To make the oatmeal, put the oats and wheat germ, if using, into a saucepan with the milk. Bring to a boil, stirring occasionally. Reduce the heat and simmer, stirring frequently, for 7 minutes until smooth and creamy.
3 Spoon the oatmeal into two bowls, top with a spoonful of apricot sauce or mix the purée in to give a swirly effect. Top with a spoonful of honey and a sprinkling of linseeds, if desired.

DATE & VANILLA ENERGY SPREAD

This makes a healthier, low-sugar alternative to commercially made jams, which by their nature are high in sugar and, with cheaper brands, low in fruit content. A spoonful of this rich spread is delicious on a whole wheat English muffin. It can also be served with yogurt, oatmeal, or as a filling in pancakes.

1½ cups chopped dried dates
1 cup water
1 tsp vanilla extract

1 Place the dates and water in a heavy-based saucepan. Bring to a boil, then reduce the heat and simmer, covered, for 20 minutes until the fruit is tender and most of the water has been absorbed.
2 Transfer to a food processor or blender and add the vanilla extract; purée until smooth. Set aside to cool and store in an airtight container in the refrigerator, where the spread will keep for up to a week.

SUNNYSIDE-UP BREAKFAST

This nifty breakfast catches the imagination of children and is perfect brain fuel for the day ahead, being a nutritious combination of protein and carbohydrates. Broiled tomatoes or baked beans add the finishing touch!

Serves 1

1 slice seeded whole wheat bread
butter, for spreading
1 egg
broiled tomatoes or baked beans,
    to serve

1 Preheat the broiler to high. Stamp out a circle, about 2 inches in diameter, in the center of the slice of bread using a cookie cutter.
2 Line the broiler pan with foil. Toast one side of the bread. Turn the bread over, spread the top with butter, and break the egg into the hole in the center. Broil for 3–5 minutes until just set.
3 Using a spatula, carefully lift the toast and egg together and transfer to a serving plate. Serve immediately with broiled tomatoes or baked beans.

POTATO PANCAKES WITH BACON

A great way of using up leftover mashed potatoes, these savory mini potato pancakes are equally good served with broiled tomatoes, good-quality sausages, or baked beans, or drizzled with maple syrup, if desired.

Serves 4

scant ½ cup cold mashed potatoes
scant 1 cup milk
⅔ cup whole wheat all-purpose flour
pinch of salt
1 egg, beaten
sunflower oil, for frying
good-quality bacon, broiled until crisp,
    to serve
broiled tomatoes, to serve (optional)
maple syrup, to serve (optional)

1 Blend the mashed potatoes and milk in a food processor or blender to make a thin potato purée.
2 Put the flour and salt in a bowl, make a well in the center of the flour and add the beaten egg, then gradually add the potato purée. Beat to make a smooth, fairly thick batter.
3 Heat a little oil in a large nonstick frying pan. Place a small ladleful of batter per cake into the pan – you will probably need to work in batches. Cook each pancake for 2 minutes on each side until golden. Keep the cooked potato cakes warm as you cook.
4 Divide the pancakes between the four plates, add a slice of bacon and broiled tomatoes, or drizzle with maple syrup if using.

BUBBLE "N" SQUEAK PATTIES

Cabbage is not always a favorite with children. Here, it is crisp and partly disguised by the cheesy mashed potatoes. Serve with low-sugar and low-salt baked beans.

Makes 6 patties
½ cup Savoy cabbage, very finely
   shredded
1 heaping cup cold mashed potatoes
½ cup sharp Cheddar cheese, grated
1 tsp Dijon mustard
salt and pepper, to taste

1 small egg, beaten
flour, for coating
sunflower oil, for frying

1 Steam the cabbage for 3 minutes until just tender. Leave to cool and squeeze with your hands to remove as much water as possible.
2 Mix the cabbage with the mashed potatoes, cheese, and mustard, then season to taste. Stir in the egg and mix until combined.

3 Divide the mixture into sixths and form each portion into a flat patty using floured hands. Coat each patty in flour and shake to remove any excess.
4 Lightly coat the bottom of a large heavy-based frying pan with oil. Cook three patties at a time for 3–4 minutes each side until golden. Drain on paper towels before serving.

ALL-AMERICAN FRITTATA

Kids love this complete breakfast in a pan, which is rather similar to an Italian frittata. Chopped bacon, onions, or mushrooms can be used instead of the sausage and tomatoes. This dish also makes a perfect after-school snack.

Serves 3–4
3 good-quality sausages (or vegetarian alternatives)
sunflower oil, for frying
4 cooked medium-size potatoes, cooled and cut into quarters
6 cherry tomatoes, halved

salt and pepper, to taste
3 eggs, beaten
whole wheat bread, toasted, to serve

1 Preheat the broiler to medium-high. Broil the sausages on a foil-lined broiler pan until cooked through and golden brown. Leave to cool slightly, then slice into large chunks.
2 Meanwhile, heat a little oil in a medium-size heavy-based frying pan with an ovenproof handle. Fry the potatoes until lightly golden all over, then add the tomatoes and cook for an additional 2 minutes. Arrange the sausages in the pan so there is an even distribution of potatoes, tomatoes, and sausages.
3 Add a little more oil to the pan if it seems dry. Season the beaten eggs and pour the mixture over the ingredients in the pan. Cook for 3 minutes without stirring or disturbing the omelet. Place under the preheated broiler for 3 minutes until the top is just cooked. Serve cut into wedges with whole wheat toast.

SMOKED SALMON OMELET

This may sound a bit "glam" for a children's book but it works incredibly well, and smoked salmon – or smoked trout – can be a useful way to introduce oily fish to children. Served with seeded whole wheat bread, it makes a quick weekend brunch that should be popular with the whole family.

Serves 1–2
small pat of butter
2 eggs, beaten
few strips of smoked salmon or trout
freshly ground black pepper, to serve
   (optional)

1 Melt the butter in a heavy-based, nonstick frying pan and swirl it around to coat the bottom.
2 Pour in the beaten eggs. As the omelet begins to set, push the edges toward the center, allowing the raw egg to run into the edge of the pan. Cook for about 1 minute, and when lightly set and still runny on top, arrange the smoked salmon strips on one half of the omelet. Fold the omelet in half to enclose the salmon and cook briefly.
3 Turn out onto a plate and serve, seasoned with freshly ground black pepper, if desired.

QUICK SNACKS

These tasty snacks are useful at any time of day – and the great news is that they are full of goodness, too! Children need to recharge their energy levels more often than adults, so it's a good idea to have some of these readily available.

Zinc has been directly linked to childhood intelligence and its deficiency is disturbingly common. **Beans** are a good source of this valuable mineral, while **tomatoes** are a good source of antioxidant nutrients, lycopene, vitamin C, and beta-carotene, which protect the brain and nervous system.

TOMATO & BEAN DIP

Spread on whole grain crackers, whole wheat bread or English muffins, this creamy dip makes a nutritious snack.

About 10 servings
3 vine-ripened tomatoes, quartered
   and seeded
3 garlic cloves, left whole in their skin
2 tbsp omega-blend or extra-virgin
   olive oil
7-oz can cannellini beans, drained and
   rinsed
2 tbsp fresh lemon juice
salt and pepper, to taste

1 Preheat the oven to 400°F. Place the tomatoes and garlic in a roasting pan and coat with 1 tbsp oil. Roast for 15 minutes until the garlic is soft and the tomatoes tender.
2 Peel the garlic, skin the tomatoes, and place in a food processor or blender with the remaining oil, the beans, and lemon juice. Purée until smooth and season to taste. Store in the refrigerator in an airtight container (keeps for up to a week).

AVOCADO DIP

Crunchy raw vegetables seem to be more acceptable to many children, and dipping them into this nutritious garlicky guacamole adds to the appeal.

Serves 2–4
1 ripe medium-size avocado
1 small garlic clove, crushed
1 tbsp lemon juice
1 tbsp mayonnaise
various raw vegetables, such as
   broccoli, cauliflower, bell peppers,
   cucumber, celery, baby corn, carrots,
   snow peas

1 Cut the avocado in half and remove the pit. Scoop the flesh out of the skin. Transfer the flesh to a blender or processor and add the garlic, lemon juice, and mayonnaise. Process until the dip is the consistency you prefer. Alternatively, place the ingredients in a bowl and mash together.
2 Prepare the vegetables to dip into the avocado mixture: cut broccoli and cauliflower into florets; de-seed the peppers and cut into strips; cut celery, cucumber, and carrots into sticks, and leave snow peas and baby corn whole. You may wish to blanche the snow peas or corn slightly first. Serve with the dip.

Although **avocados** are fairly high in fat, it is the beneficial mono-unsaturated type. Avocados are best eaten when just ripe to get the full benefit of their antioxidant vitamins A, C, and E, which protect brain cells against destructive free radicals. They also contain B-complex vitamins for memory and clarity of thought.

NUT & SEED SNACK

Potato chips contain high amounts of the wrong type of fat, namely saturated, as well as salt and often unwanted additives. This soy-flavored mixed nut and seed snack makes a nutritious alternative. However, go easy on the soy sauce, as it is very salty – only a little is needed to add flavor.

Serves 2

1 cup mixed unsalted raw nuts and seeds, such as cashews, almonds, hazelnuts, peanuts, sunflower, and pumpkin seeds

1 tsp soy sauce

WARNING

Children under five should not be given whole nuts because of the danger of choking. If there is a history of peanut allergy in the family or you are concerned about allergies, consult your doctor before giving nuts to children.

1 Preheat the oven to 225°F. Rub any papery brown skins off the peanuts, if using. Place all the nuts on a baking sheet and roast for 10 minutes, until just golden.
2 Add the seeds and mix well. Cook for an additional 5 minutes until slightly brown. Add the soy sauce to the nuts and seeds and toss well to coat.

NUT & SEED BUTTER

Read the labels of many commercial peanut butters and you will find sugar, palm oil, salt, and preservatives, often in significant amounts. Homemade alternatives are quick and simple to make – and you choose the ingredients. This version uses a cold-pressed omega-blend oil that incorporates brain-boosting omega-3, -6, and -9. Find it in health food shops and in some supermarkets in the special diet section.

About 10 servings

scant ⅓ cup unsalted cashews

scant ⅓ cup blanched almonds

scant ⅓ cup unsalted peanuts

1 tbsp pumpkin seeds

1 tbsp sunflower seeds

3 tbsp omega-blend or sunflower oil

1–2 tbsp olive oil

½ tsp salt

1 Lightly toast the nuts and seeds in a dry frying pan over medium-high heat for 3 minutes, stirring frequently, until golden. Leave to cool and remove the papery brown covering from any peanuts, if necessary.
2 Place the toasted nuts and seeds, oils, and salt in a food processor and blend until fairly smooth and creamy. Transfer to a jar and store in the refrigerator.

COOL DOGS

A nifty alternative to the high-fat, often poor-quality hot dog, the cool dog is made using good-quality sausages and a warm soft tortilla – simple and quick! This is a good example of a meal that is as good as its ingredients. Use the best sausages that you can find and you won't be filling your children with unwanted additives. And if you're using store-bought bottled sauces to serve, look out for the "no added sugar and salt" varieties.

RED PEPPER HUMMUS

Hummus is far more versatile than its usual use as a dip. It also makes a nutritious addition to soups, stews, and pasta sauces. The roasted red pepper in this recipe adds a delicious smoky sweetness as well as the beneficial antioxidants vitamin C and beta-carotene.

About 10 servings
1 small red bell pepper, de-seeded and
   cut into thick strips
3 tbsp extra-virgin olive oil
8-oz can "no added salt and sugar"
   garbanzo beans, drained and rinsed
2 garlic cloves, crushed
1 tbsp light tahini (sesame seed paste)
1 tbsp warm water
juice of ½ lemon
salt and pepper, to taste

1 Preheat the oven to 400°F. Place the red pepper in a roasting pan with 1 tbsp oil and mix well to ensure the pepper is completely coated. Roast for 35–40 minutes until tender and the skin begins to blister. Transfer the pepper to a plastic bag or wrap in foil, and leave to cool. When the pepper is cool enough to handle, remove from the bag or foil and rub off the skin.
2 Place the pepper strips, garbanzos, garlic, tahini, water, lemon juice, and remaining oil in a food processor or blender and purée until smooth. Season to taste.

Serves 2
4 good-quality pork sausages or
   vegetarian alternative
1 small soft flour tortilla, cut into
   4 strips
mayonnaise, ketchup, guacamole, or
   hummus, to serve

1 Preheat the broiler to medium-high. Line a broiler pan with foil and arrange the sausages on top. Broil the sausages until cooked through and golden.
2 Place the tortilla strips in a dry frying pan and heat until warmed through. When the sausages are cooked, lay them on the tortilla strips, add some mayonnaise, ketchup, guacamole, or hummus and serve.

BRAIN BOX

Garbanzo beans provide a good mix of brain-enhancing minerals, including magnesium, phosphorus, zinc, and manganese, necessary for constructing the brain's messengers.

TUNA TORTILLA MELT

Soft, floury tortillas are perfect for filling with all sorts of healthy goodies. If you can find whole wheat versions, all the better. You could also use whole wheat pita bread for this.

Serves 1–2
½ cup canned tuna in spring
  water or olive oil, drained
1 large soft tortilla
¼ cup grated sharp Cheddar cheese
1 small tomato, sliced

BRAIN BOX

Tuna is one of the oily fish family providing omega-3 fats, essential for brain development and function. Although the canned variety is lower in these beneficial oils than fresh tuna, it still makes a convenient protein food.

---

1 Mash the drained tuna with a fork and arrange it in the center of the tortilla. Top with the grated Cheddar and sliced tomato.
2 Roll up the tortilla to enclose the filling. Heat a dry, nonstick frying pan over medium heat. Place the tortilla seam-side down in the pan and cook for 3 minutes until warmed through and golden. Cut in half diagonally and serve.

GET-SMART TOASTIES

Fresh sardines are very bony, so they tend not to be popular with children, but the tinned variety is a useful alternative. Here, they are mixed with fresh tomato and pesto to dilute the fishy flavor.

Serves 2
2 slices whole wheat bread
1 can boneless sardines in tomato
  sauce
1 heaping tbsp red pesto
1 tomato, de-seeded and chopped

1 Preheat the broiler to medium-high. Line a broiler pan with foil. Cut one slice of bread into a fish shape either freehand or using a cookie cutter, incorporating as much of the bread as possible to reduce wastage. Repeat with the other slice of bread.
2 Mash the sardines and mix with the pesto and tomato.

3 Toast one side of each fish-shaped piece of bread, then turn over and lightly toast the other side. Spoon the sardine mixture on top and broil for 3 minutes until heated through.

BRAIN BOX

Oily fish, such as **canned sardines**, provide beneficial brainboosting oils, which have been found to increase brain capacity, improving memory and concentration.

FRENCH TOAST

Also known as "eggy bread," French toast works just as well when made with fruit bread or brioche and makes a quick comforting snack.

Serves 2
2 slices whole wheat bread
1 egg, beaten, mixed with 2 tbsp milk
2 tbsp unsalted butter

Dip each slice of bread into the egg-and-milk mixture until evenly covered. Melt the butter in a heavy-based frying pan and add the egg-soaked bread. Cook for 1–2 minutes on each side until the egg has set and the toast is golden brown.

PIZZA POWER

All kids love pizza, and homemade versions offer a good range of nutrients. This speedy recipe is perfect for hungry tummies that need to be filled in next to no time.

Serves 2
2 whole wheat English muffins, halved
4 tsp red pesto
1 tomato, de-seeded and chopped
4 slices mozzarella

1 Preheat the broiler to medium-high. Line a broiler pan with foil. Lightly toast the uncut side of each muffin half.
2 Mix together the pesto and tomato and spoon on top of the untoasted side of each muffin half. Top with the mozzarella cheese and return to the broiler for 3–5 minutes until melted and bubbling. Leave to cool slightly before serving.

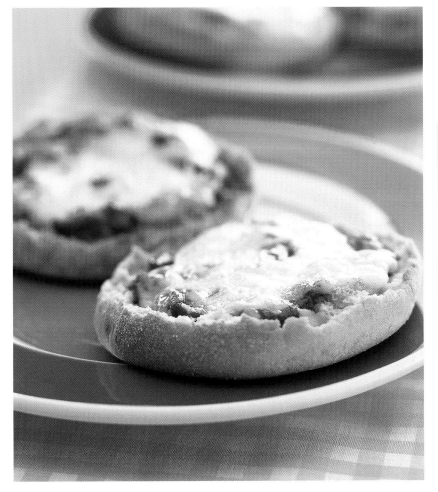

BRAIN BOX

Mozzarella cheese is a valuable low-fat protein food which, when combined with the muffins (a source of complex carbohydrate), will provide plenty of long-term energy.

MAIN DISHES

The recipes found in this section are perfect for weekday meals when your time in the kitchen may be limited. Full of goodness and very tasty, they will appeal to children and adults alike.

MIGHTY MINESTRONE

This adaptation of the popular Italian soup contains a multitude of beneficial brain foods from vegetables and beans to pasta and cheese. It tastes even better when made in advance. Serve with slices of garlic bread to boost carbohydrate intake.

Serves 4

2 tbsp olive oil
1 leek, sliced
1 carrot, finely chopped
1 stalk celery, finely chopped
3 green beans, finely sliced
1 quart vegetable bouillon
1¼ cups tomato purée
2 bay leaves
scant 1 cup pasta shapes, e.g., shells
⅔ cup canned cannellini beans,
   drained and rinsed
sprig of fresh rosemary
salt and pepper, to taste
freshly grated Parmesan cheese,
   to serve

1 Heat the oil in a large heavy-based saucepan over medium heat and add the leek. Cook for 5 minutes, stirring occasionally, until tender. Add the carrot, celery, and green beans and cook for an additional 5 minutes.
2 Pour in the bouillon and tomato purée and add the bay leaves; stir well. Bring to a boil, then reduce the heat and simmer, half-covered, for 15 minutes. Remove and reserve the bay

| BRAIN | BOX |

Beans contain B-complex vitamins, iron, zinc, and magnesium, all of which are vital for brain function, memory, and a healthy nervous system.

leaves and, using a hand blender (or food processor), purée the vegetables slightly, so that there are still some bits of vegetable in the soup.
3 Return the bay leaves to the soup, add the pasta, beans, and rosemary and bring to a boil. Reduce the heat slightly and cook for 10 minutes or until the pasta is tender. Remove the bay leaves and rosemary and season to taste. You may need to add extra bouillon or water if the soup seems too thick.
4 Divide between four bowls and serve with a sprinkling of Parmesan cheese.

TOMATO & LENTIL SOUP

Tomato soup is a perennial favorite but shop-bought versions contain a surprising amount of fat, sugar, and salt, and the canning process depletes vital nutrients. This nutritious homemade version features the added health benefit of lentils and doesn't take ages to make. Serve with chunks of crusty bread.

BRAIN BOX

Recent research shows that lycopene, the pigment that turns tomatoes red, is a powerful antioxidant, protecting the brain and nervous system from destructive free radicals. Luckily, **cooked tomatoes** are just as nutritious as fresh ones.

Lentils contain the important brain combo of iron, B-complex vitamins, and zinc.

Serves 4
¼ cup dried split red lentils, rinsed
1 tbsp olive oil
1 onion, chopped
1 carrot, finely chopped
1 stick celery, finely chopped
2 cups tomato purée
2 cups vegetable bouillon
1 bay leaf
salt and pepper, to taste
3 tbsp milk

1 Place the lentils in a saucepan, cover with water, and bring to a boil. Reduce the heat and simmer, half-covered, for 15 minutes or until just tender. Using a slotted spoon, remove any scum that rises to the surface. Drain the lentils well and set aside.

2 Meanwhile, heat the oil in a large heavy-based saucepan over medium heat. Add the onion, cover the pan, and sweat for 8 minutes or until softened and transparent. Add the carrot and celery, cover, and cook for an additional 3 minutes, stirring occasionally to prevent the vegetables from sticking to the bottom of the pan.

3 Add the tomato purée, bouillon, lentils, and bay leaf. Bring to a boil. Reduce the heat and simmer, half-covered, for 25 minutes or until the lentils and vegetables are tender and the soup has thickened.

4 Carefully pour the soup into a blender or use a hand blender to purée until smooth. Return to the pan, season to taste, and stir in the milk. Reheat if necessary, and serve.

CHICKEN NOODLE SOUP

If time is short, this nutritious miso soup is just the thing. It's simple to make and contains calm-inducing carbohydrates in the form of noodles and protein-rich mini chicken dumplings. You can find packets of miso soup in health food shops and some supermarkets.

Serves 2
scant 1 cup medium egg noodles
1 medium-size bok choy, halved
2 packets instant miso soup
2 tsp soy sauce
1 small carrot, cut into fine sticks
1 scallion, cut into fine slivers
sesame seeds, for sprinkling

for the chicken dumplings:
⅔ cup ground raw chicken
1 small egg
½ tsp cornstarch
½ tsp paprika
1 tsp ground coriander
1 scallion, finely chopped
salt and pepper, to taste

BRAIN BOX

Miso soup is made from a mixture of soybeans and rice, wheat, or barley. It has a cleansing, rejuvenating effect on the body, helping it to get rid of toxins that can cloud the brain.

Chicken is a high-protein food that helps to focus the mind.

1 To make the chicken dumplings, combine the ingredients in a bowl until well mixed. Bring a pan of water to a boil. Using two teaspoons, form the chicken mixture into small balls, then drop them into the boiling water. Poach the balls, a few at a time, for 5 minutes until cooked through. Keep the cooked dumplings warm.

2 Meanwhile, cook the noodles in boiling water for about 5 minutes or until tender, adding the bok choy 2 minutes before the end of the cooking time. Drain well and slice the bok choy.

3 Dilute the miso soup according to the packet instructions. Add the soy sauce and stir well.

4 To serve, divide the noodles between two bowls, then pour in the miso soup. Stir in the bok choy, carrot, and scallion. Sprinkle with the sesame seeds and arrange the chicken dumplings on top.

POTATO NESTS

The carbohydrates provided by the potatoes help to boost levels of serotonin, the brain-calming chemical – making this a perfect meal for the end of the day. An egg nestles in the center of each potato ring for extra goodness. Serve with a green vegetable of your choice.

Serves 2
10 oz new potatoes, halved
1 large carrot, cut into three pieces
salt and pepper, to taste
sunflower oil, for frying
2 eggs

1 Steam the potatoes and carrot for 10 minutes until just tender but not completely cooked. Leave to cool, then peel the potatoes and coarsely grate them and the carrot into a bowl.

2 Season the potato mixture and divide in half. Shape each half into a ring with a hole in the center – they are quite fragile but will firm up when cooked.

3 Preheat the broiler to medium. Pour enough oil to just cover the bottom of a heavy-based frying pan and warm over medium-high heat. Carefully place the potato rings in the pan and cook for 7 minutes on one side until golden, then turn them over and cook for an additional 5 minutes. Break an egg into the hole in the center of each nest and cook for an additional 2 minutes.

4 Place the frying pan under the preheated broiler and cook the potato nests for another 2 minutes or until the egg is just set, and serve.

EGGS FLORENTINE

It can be a challenge to encourage children to eat green vegetables, but here the creamy sauce helps to make the spinach more palatable. Serve this dish with pasta, rice, or bread.

Serves 2
4¼ cups young leaf spinach, washed and rinsed well
3 tbsp heavy cream or sour cream
a little grated nutmeg
2 eggs
⅓ cup grated sharp Cheddar cheese

1 Steam the spinach for a few minutes until tender. Leave to drain, then squeeze out any excess water using your hands. Finely chop the spinach, then mix with the cream and a little grated nutmeg in a small pan and cook until heated through. Spoon the spinach into a small ovenproof dish.
2 Make two holes in the spinach mixture, large enough to accommodate the eggs. Break the eggs into the holes, top with the grated cheese, and broil for 2–3 minutes until the eggs have set.

BRAIN BOX

B-complex vitamins found in **eggs** are essential for optimum brain functioning, particularly clarity of thought.

The vitamin C in the **spinach** helps the absorption of the iron also found in this green vegetable. Iron helps boost energy levels.

HIGH-ENERGY BEAN BURGERS

Cheap meat-based burgers offer little in the way of nourishment and are high in fat and additives. These veggie versions take a little more effort but provide numerous health benefits.

Makes 4 burgers
scant ⅔ cup canned kidney beans, drained and rinsed
½ onion, grated
1 small carrot, grated
⅔ cup fresh whole wheat bread crumbs
1 tbsp smooth peanut butter
1 egg, beaten
salt and pepper, to taste
flour, for coating
sunflower oil, for frying
4 whole wheat hamburger buns or seeded bagels, to serve
shredded lettuce, tomato, and cucumber slices, to serve

1 Put the kidney beans in a food processor or blender with the onion, carrot, bread crumbs, peanut butter, and egg. Blend until the mixture forms a coarse purée. Season, then chill for 1 hour to allow the mixture to firm up.
2 Form the mixture into four burgers using floured hands, then dip each burger into flour to coat.
3 Heat enough oil to just cover the bottom of a large, heavy-based frying pan. Cook the burgers, two at a time, for about 3 minutes on each side or until golden and crisp. Drain on paper towels. Repeat with the remaining burgers. (To broil the burgers, brush with oil and broil for about 4 minutes on each side.)
4 To serve, split each hamburger bun or bagel in half. Add the burgers and lettuce, tomato, and cucumber, as desired. Serve with a spoonful of hummus, guacamole, or tomato ketchup.

DREAMY CHINESE RICE

Parents will welcome this lightly spiced rice dish. Brown rice is a complex carbohydrate and as such will instill feelings of sleepiness and calmness – well, that's the theory! The rice is topped with strips of omelet.

Serves 2

2 tsp sunflower oil
splash of toasted sesame oil
1 garlic clove, chopped
½ tsp Chinese five-spice powder
¼ red bell pepper, de-seeded and diced
4 baby corn, cut into coins
4 small broccoli florets
1 scallion, sliced diagonally
small knob of fresh gingerroot, peeled
     and grated (optional)
¼ cup fresh apple juice
2 tbsp bouillon or water
scant 2 cups cold, cooked brown rice
2 tsp soy sauce
1 tsp sesame seeds

for the omelet:
small pat of butter
1 egg, beaten

1 Heat the sunflower and sesame oils in a wok or heavy-based frying pan. Add the garlic, Chinese five spice powder, red bell pepper, baby corn, broccoli, scallion, and ginger (if using) and stir-fry for 4 minutes.

2 Add the apple juice and water and stir-fry for another 3 minutes or until the vegetables are tender.

3 Add the rice and soy sauce to the wok and stir until thoroughly warmed through. Mix in the sesame seeds.

4 To make the omelet, melt the butter in a small frying pan and add the egg. Swirl the egg until it covers the base of the pan. Cook until the egg has set, then turn out onto a plate. Cut into strips.

5 To serve, divide the rice between two bowls and arrange the omelet strips on top.

> ### WARNING
>
> It is important to make sure that the **cooked rice** has been heated through thoroughly before serving. Cooked rice that has been reheated inadequately is a surprisingly common source of food poisoning.

NICE RICE & VEGGIE FRITTERS

These are easy to prepare and make use of leftover brown rice. Serve them with low-sugar and low-salt baked beans or steamed green vegetables.

BRAIN BOX

Complex carbohydrates (here in **brown rice**) have a soothing effect on the mind since they stimulate the release of the calming chemical serotonin in the brain. They also provide plenty of long-term energy, keeping blood sugar levels steady, which is important for a good night's sleep. Brown rice also contains B-complex vitamins, essential for healthy brain function.

Makes 8 fritters

heaping ⅔ cup cold cooked brown rice
1 small leek, finely chopped
½ yellow bell pepper, de-seeded and finely diced
1 garlic clove, crushed
2 tbsp freshly grated Parmesan cheese
1 small egg, beaten
2 tbsp heavy cream
2 tbsp flour
salt and pepper, to taste
sunflower oil, for frying

1 Mix together the rice, leek, yellow bell pepper, garlic, Parmesan cheese, egg, cream, and flour in a bowl to make a sloppy batter. Season to taste.
2 Heat enough oil to lightly coat the bottom of a heavy-based frying pan. Place one heaping tablespoon of the rice mixture per fritter into the hot oil and flatten slightly with a spatula. Cook in batches for 3 minutes on each side until golden. Drain on paper towels before serving.

VEGETABLE & TOFU KEBABS
WITH A SATAY DIP

A powerhouse of brain nutrients are provided by these colorful vegetable kebabs, which are served with a peanut dipping sauce. These kebabs also make a good vegetarian addition – for children or adults – to a barbecue. Serve with a warm tortilla or pita bread. The satay dip will keep for up to a week if stored in the refrigerator.

Makes 4 kebabs
5 oz tofu (bean curd), cut into 8 cubes
2 zucchini, cut into 8 chunks
4 cherry tomatoes
¼ yellow bell pepper, cut into 4 chunks

for the marinade:
1 tbsp honey
1 tsp soy sauce
1 tbsp toasted sesame oil
1 tsp olive oil
1 garlic clove, sliced

for the satay dip:
2 tbsp smooth peanut butter
1 tsp olive oil
1 tsp hot water
1 tsp soy sauce
½ tsp light brown sugar
2 tbsp mayonnaise

1 To make the marinade, mix the ingredients together in a shallow nonmetallic dish. Put the tofu, zucchini, cherry tomatoes, and bell pepper in the marinade. Cover with plastic wrap and leave to marinate for at least 1 hour or preferably overnight, turning the vegetables and tofu occasionally.
2 Place four wooden skewers in a bowl of water and leave to soak for 30 minutes – this helps to prevent the skewers from burning. Meanwhile, to make the dip, combine the ingredients in a small bowl and mix together well.
3 Preheat the broiler to medium-high. Line the broiler pan with foil. Arrange the tofu and vegetables on the soaked skewers, reserving the marinade: place a piece of zucchini, then a tofu cube, a

BRAIN BOX

Vitamin C found in **bell peppers, tomatoes, and zucchini** aids the absorption of minerals such as iron.

Tofu (bean curd) is a low-fat protein, rich in minerals, particularly iron, magnesium, and calcium, important nutrients for a healthy nervous system and brain.

cherry tomato, chunk of pepper, another tofu cube, and finally another piece of zucchini on each skewer. Repeat to make three more kebabs.

4 Arrange the kebabs on the broiler pan. Brush with the reserved marinade. Broil for 8–10 minutes, turning occasionally and brushing with the marinade, until golden. Serve with the satay dip.

QUICK TOMATO PASTA

Encouraging children to eat vegetables is an ongoing challenge, and while it's important to promote a love of vegetables, attempts don't always work. This pasta sauce – with its sneaky hidden vegetables – is very popular with my kids.

Serves 2
4 oz whole wheat spaghetti
freshly grated Parmesan cheese,
   to serve

for the sauce:
1 tbsp olive oil
1 small onion, finely chopped
½ red bell pepper, de-seeded and diced
1 large garlic clove, crushed
1 tsp dried oregano
1 carrot, finely chopped
1¼ cups tomato purée
1 tsp tomato paste
¼ tsp superfine sugar (optional)
salt and pepper, to taste

1 Heat the oil in a medium-size heavy-based saucepan over medium heat and cook the onion for 7 minutes, half-covered, or until softened. Add the red bell pepper and cook for an additional 3 minutes, half-covered, stirring frequently. Add the garlic and oregano and cook for 1 minute. Meanwhile, steam the carrot for 5 minutes until just tender.

2 Pour in the tomato purée, then stir in the tomato paste, sugar (if using), and carrot, season and cook for about 8 minutes over low heat until reduced and thickened. Purée the sauce in a food processor until smooth and creamy.

3 Meanwhile, cook the pasta following the package instructions. Drain, reserving 2 tablespoons of the cooking water. Combine the pasta, cooking liquid, and sauce. Serve sprinkled with Parmesan cheese.

BACON & PEA PENNE

Try to buy good-quality Canadian bacon for the best flavor and health benefits. For extra goodness serve this dish with steamed broccoli.

Serves 2
2 slices Canadian bacon
1 cup uncooked penne pasta
1 tbsp olive oil
1 large garlic clove, chopped
½ cup vegetable bouillon
¾ cup frozen peas
3 tbsp sour cream
salt and pepper, to taste
freshly grated Parmesan cheese,
   to serve

1 Broil the bacon until crisp. Cook the pasta in boiling water following the package instructions. Drain, reserving about 1 tablespoon of the cooking water.
2 Meanwhile, heat the olive oil in a heavy-based frying pan over medium-high heat and fry the garlic for 1 minute or until softened. Add the bouillon and the peas and cook for 2 minutes or until the peas are cooked and the liquid has reduced.
3 Cut the bacon into small pieces and add to the pan with the sour cream. Cook over low heat, stirring frequently, until warmed through. Stir the pasta and reserved water into the sauce and mix gently until combined. Season to taste and serve sprinkled with cheese.

BRAIN BOX

Peas are little nuggets of goodness, providing plenty of vitamin C and B-complex vitamins as well as zinc, a nutrient that aids concentration. This even applies to frozen peas, which can be more nutritious than fresh, if the latter have been stored for some time.

Canadian bacon also provides B vitamins, essential for the health of the nervous system.

SALMON KEBABS

The marinade gives these salmon kebabs a wonderful sweet, glossy glaze. A certain amount of forward planning is required, as they need to marinate for at least an hour to absorb the flavors of the marinade. While kebabs are fun, do take care with the skewers when giving them to children. They are served with a fruity couscous, and you can add a green vegetable for extra health benefits.

Serves 2
5 oz skinless salmon fillet, cut into
   16 cubes

for the marinade:
1 tbsp honey
2 tsp soy sauce
1 tsp omega-blend oil or olive oil
1 tsp toasted sesame oil
1 garlic clove, sliced

for the fruity couscous:
¼ cup couscous
vegetable bouillon, for soaking
small pat of butter
½ nectarine or peach, diced
1 tbsp toasted sesame seeds
1 tbsp toasted flaked almonds

1 Mix together the ingredients for the marinade in a shallow, nonmetallic dish. Add the cubes of salmon and turn until the fish is coated in the marinade. Cover with plastic wrap and leave to marinate in the refrigerator for at least 1 hour, preferably overnight, turning the fish occasionally.
2 To make the couscous, pour the couscous grains into a heatproof bowl. Bring the vegetable bouillon to a boil and pour enough into the bowl to just

cover the couscous – there should be about ¼ in bouillon above the couscous. Let stand until the grains have absorbed all of the liquid. Add a small pat of butter and fluff up with a fork. Stir in the diced nectarine, seeds, and nuts and set aside.

3 Meanwhile, soak four wooden skewers in a bowl of water for 30 minutes to prevent them from burning. Preheat the broiler to high and line the broiler pan with foil. Thread the cubes of salmon onto the skewers and brush with the marinade. Broil the kebabs for 3–5 minutes, turning halfway through and brushing with more marinade, until cooked through. Serve with the fruity couscous.

FANTASTIC FAJITAS

Add a taste of Mexico to mealtimes with these healthy shrimp-filled tortillas. Serve with a green salad or chunks of bell pepper, carrot, and cucumber to dip into creamy avocado dip (see page 57) or red pepper hummus (see page 59).

Serves 2
1 tbsp olive oil
1 garlic clove, chopped
½ red bell pepper, de-seeded and cut into strips
⅔ cup tomato purée
½ tsp ground cumin
1 tbsp tomato paste
juice of ½ lime
4 oz cooked shrimp, defrosted if frozen

BRAIN BOX

Shrimp contain an amino acid called tyrosine, which helps to increase alertness, as well as zinc, a crucial brain mineral that helps to control mood swings and irritability.

2 small soft tortillas
½ small avocado, pitted, peeled, and diced, to serve
spoonfuls of sour cream or yogurt with live and active cultures, to serve

1 Heat the olive oil in a heavy-based frying pan over a medium-low heat and fry the garlic and red bell pepper for 3 minutes until softened. Add the tomato purée, cumin, and tomato paste and cook for 8 minutes over a medium heat until reduced and thickened. Add the lime juice and stir in the shrimp; heat well.

2 Warm the tortillas, then spoon the shrimp mixture on one side of each one. Top the filling with the diced avocado and spoon the sour cream or yogurt on top. Fold the tortillas over to enclose the filling and serve.

SALMON FINGERS WITH SWEET POTATO FRIES

This healthy version of the children's classic fish fingers and French fries offers plenty of mind-stimulating nutrients. If making your own sounds a bit daunting, be reassured that these salmon fingers are quick and easy to make. Peas are a must as an accompaniment.

Serves 2–3
7 oz skinless salmon fillet
¾ cup fine cornmeal or polenta
2 tbsp freshly grated Parmesan cheese
1 egg, beaten
sunflower oil, for frying
salt and pepper, to taste

for the sweet potato fries:
1 small sweet potato, scrubbed and cut into wedges
2 tsp olive oil

1 Preheat the oven to 400°F. To make the fries, dry the sweet potatoes on a clean kitchen towel. Spoon the oil into a roasting pan and heat briefly. Toss the sweet potatoes in the warm oil until coated and roast for 30 minutes, turning them halfway through, until tender and golden.
2 Meanwhile, cut the salmon into six thick finger shapes. Mix together the cornmeal or polenta and Parmesan cheese on a plate. Dip each salmon finger into the beaten egg, then roll in the cornmeal and Parmesan mixture until evenly coated.
3 Pour enough oil into a large heavy-based frying pan to cover the base and warm over medium-high heat.
4 Carefully arrange the salmon fingers in the pan and cook for 6 minutes, turning halfway through, until golden. Drain on paper towels, season, then serve with the sweet potato fries.

BRAIN BOX

Sweet potatoes, particularly the orange-fleshed variety, provide the antioxidants vitamin C and beta-carotene, which help to enhance memory.

SUPER FISH!

This simple fish supper couldn't be easier to make but looks great – and for those kids who are not big fans of fish, the mozzarella, pesto, and tomato topping adds plenty of color and flavor. Serve with new potatoes and corn on the cob.

Serves 2
2 5-oz skinless cod fillets
olive oil, for brushing
2 heaping tsp red or green pesto
1 tomato, sliced and de-seeded
2 slices mozzarella cheese
salt and pepper, to taste

1 Preheat the broiler to high and line a broiler pan with foil. Check the cod for any remaining bones and remove. Brush both sides of each fillet with the oil. Place the fish in the broiler pan and broil for 3 minutes; turn and cook for an additional 2–3 minutes until opaque and just cooked through.
2 Remove the pan from the broiler and arrange a heaping spoonful of pesto on top of each fillet. Arrange the tomato slices and the mozzarella on top of the pesto. Broil for 3–4 minutes until the mozzarella has melted and is turning slightly golden. Season and serve.

EASY-PEASY FISH PIE

This fish pie packs a powerful punch when it comes to brain-nurturing nutrients. It cuts a few corners when it comes to preparation in that it gets its creaminess from sour cream rather than a white sauce. Steamed broccoli or green beans go particularly well with this dish.

Serves 2

8 oz skinless cod fillet
3 oz undyed skinless smoked haddock
  fillet
milk, for poaching
2 tsp olive oil
1 garlic clove, chopped
1 small leek, sliced
¾ cup frozen peas
scant ½ cup low-fat sour cream
1 tsp Dijon mustard
1 tbsp snipped fresh chives
1 egg, hard-boiled and quartered

for the mashed potatoes:
1 lb potatoes, peeled and cut
  into chunks
1 tbsp olive oil
2 tbsp butter
¼ cup warm milk or the milk used to
  poach the fish
salt and pepper, to taste

1 To make the mashed potatoes, cook the potatoes in boiling water for 15–20 minutes until tender. Drain well.
2 Meanwhile, place the fish in a frying pan and just cover with milk. Poach the fish for 8 minutes or until just cooked. Remove the fish from the poaching liquid and flake into large chunks, removing any stray bones.

3 Heat 2 tsp oil in a large heavy-based frying pan and fry the garlic and leek for 5 minutes. Add the peas and cook briefly, stirring constantly. Stir in the sour cream and mustard. Cook until heated through and carefully stir in the chives, hard-boiled egg, and cooked fish. Spoon the mixture into a flameproof dish.
4 Preheat the broiler to medium. Drain the potatoes well and add the olive oil, butter, and warm milk (or fish-poaching milk). Mash until smooth and creamy and spoon over the fish. Smooth the mashed potatoes slightly and place the dish under the broiler for 3–5 minutes until the top becomes golden.

BRAIN BOX

Cod is a good source of low fat protein as well as some B-group vitamins, selenium, and vitamin E, all nutrients necessary for healthy brain function.

CHICKEN & COCONUT NOODLES

Strips of chicken top the Malaysian-inspired coconut noodles in this dish. Shrimp or lean pork make tasty, nutritious alternatives to the chicken and the selection of vegetables can be adapted to suit personal tastes.

Serves 2

6 oz skinless boneless chicken breast, cut into thin strips
1 cup uncooked medium egg noodles
1 tbsp sunflower oil
1 small leek, sliced
1 garlic clove, chopped
¼ red bell pepper, de-seeded and diced
1 small zucchini, diced
4 baby corn, sliced lengthwise
6 snow peas
1 tsp mild curry powder
⅔ cup coconut milk
scant ½ cup vegetable bouillon
sesame seeds and sliced scallions, to serve (optional)

1 Preheat the broiler to high and line the broiler pan with foil. Brush the chicken with a little of the oil and broil for 8 minutes or until golden and cooked through; keep warm.
2 While the chicken is being broiled, cook the noodles according to the package instructions. Drain well and rinse under cold running water to prevent them from cooking further. Leave to drain thoroughly.
3 Heat the remaining oil in a wok and stir-fry the leek, garlic, red bell pepper, zucchini, baby corn, and snow peas for 5 minutes, tossing the vegetables frequently. Add the curry powder and cook for another minute.

BRAIN BOX

Chicken is high in good-quality protein as well as selenium, zinc, and B-complex vitamins. The skin is full of saturated fat, so it is important to remove it. Buy organic poultry if you can to avoid unwanted chemicals that may affect brain efficiency.

4 Add the coconut milk and bouillon and cook for 5 minutes or until the liquid has reduced and thickened. Add the noodles to heat through.
5 To serve, spoon the noodles, veggies, and sauce into bowls, top with the chicken strips, and sprinkle with sesame seeds and scallions, if desired.

GREAT BALLS OF...CHICKEN!

A great Italian-inspired dish that's popular with kids. Serve it with pasta or rice and a green vegetable or salad.

Serves 2
½ pound ground raw chicken
2 tbsp freshly grated Parmesan cheese
½ cup fresh bread crumbs
1 small egg, beaten
salt and pepper, to taste
sunflower oil, for frying

for the tomato sauce:
1 garlic clove, crushed
½ tsp dried oregano
1¼ cups tomato purée
pinch of sugar

1 To make the meatballs, mix together the chicken, Parmesan cheese, bread crumbs, and egg. Season lightly and, using 2 soup spoons, form into 10 small balls – they don't have to be perfectly round.
2 Heat enough oil to just cover the bottom of a heavy-based frying pan and cook the meatballs for 6–8 minutes, turning occasionally, until golden and cooked though. Remove from the pan and keep warm.
3 To make the sauce, put the garlic and oregano in the pan, adding a little more oil if necessary. Fry for 1 minute, then add the tomato purée and a pinch of sugar. Cook for 4 minutes over a medium-low heat, stirring occasionally.

4 Return the chicken balls to the pan and cook for an additional 4 minutes or until heated through and the sauce has reduced and thickened.

MAGIC BEEF WITH APRICOTS

This mildly spiced ground beef dish is magic in that it provides a potent range of essential brain nutrients from iron and beta-carotene to B-complex vitamins. Serve with a baked potato and green vegetables.

Serves 2
1 tbsp olive oil
1 small onion, finely chopped
1 garlic clove, chopped
1 small carrot, grated
½ small red bell pepper, de-seeded and diced
5 oz ground beef or vegetarian alternative
¼ tsp ground cumin
½ tsp ground cinnamon
¼ tsp ground coriander
1 cup tomato purée
½ cup chicken or vegetable bouillon
1 tbsp tomato paste
6 ready-to-eat unsulfured dried apricots
salt and pepper, to taste

1 Heat the oil in a large heavy-based saucepan over medium heat, add the onion and cook, covered, stirring occasionally, for 7 minutes or until softened and tender. Add the garlic, carrot, and bell pepper and cook, covered, for an additional 3 minutes.
2 Push the contents of the pan to one side and add the meat. Cook, uncovered, stirring frequently until browned. Stir in the spices and cook for another minute.
3 Pour in the tomato purée and bouillon and add the tomato paste and apricots. Stir well and cook, half-covered, for 30 minutes until reduced and thickened. If the sauce appears too liquid, remove the lid, or if is it too dry, add a little more bouillon. Season to taste and serve.

BRAIN BOX

Many shy away from **red meat** for various reasons, but it does have a role to play in the brain-food diet, providing all eight essential amino acids necessary to make neuro-transmitters. It is also a good source of iron, which plays a role in aiding memory and learning. Make sure you buy lean organic meat, if possible.

WEEKEND MEALS

The following recipes might take a little longer to prepare – but they are worth it!
Don't be afraid to be adventurous; the wide range of ingredients used will give
the whole family the opportunity to appreciate all sorts of different flavors.

SLEEPYTIME CHEESY PASTA

A cheese sauce can be invaluable for making vegetables more acceptable to children. Additionally, if your children are like coiled springs at the end of the day, a helping of pasta enveloped in a creamy cheese sauce may help to calm them down.

Serves 4
1½ cups penne pasta, preferably whole wheat
¾ cup broccoli florets
generous ⅓ cup cauliflower florets
1 large leek, sliced
2 tbsp butter
3 tbsp all-purpose flour
3 cups milk, warmed
1 tsp dried oregano (optional)
1 tbsp Dijon mustard
1 cup grated sharp Cheddar cheese, plus extra for sprinkling
2 tbsp fresh whole wheat bread crumbs

1 Cook the pasta in plenty of boiling salted water, following the package instructions. Meanwhile, steam the broccoli, cauliflower, and leek for 5–7 minutes until tender. Drain the pasta and transfer to a flameproof dish with the vegetables.
2 To make the cheese sauce, melt the butter in a heavy-based saucepan. Reduce the heat and stir in the flour and cook for about 2 minutes, stirring continuously with a wooden spoon

BRAIN BOX

Both **broccoli and cauliflower** belong to the cruciferous family of vegetables and provide potent antioxidants, helping to protect the brain from harmful free radicals.

until the mixture forms a thick light brown paste. Gradually add the warm milk, whisking well with a balloon whisk. Continue to add the milk and cook until the mixture has thickened and formed a silky, creamy sauce.
3 Add the oregano, if using, mustard, and cheese and heat, stirring, until the cheese has melted. Pour the sauce over the pasta and vegetables and stir gently until combined.
4 Preheat the broiler to medium-high. Sprinkle the pasta with extra grated cheese and bread crumbs and broil until the cheese has melted and the bread crumbs are golden.

BEANZ MEANZ BRAINS

Tofu is made from the highly nutritious soybean, which is rich in high-quality, low-fat protein, since it contains all eight essential amino acids. Tofu benefits from being combined with stronger flavors, as in these lightly spiced tofu cakes. They're excellent with a dollop of mango chutney, brown rice, and a salad for a light lunch or with a noodle salad (see page 82).

Makes 10 cakes
½ lb tofu, grated
1 small onion, grated
1 carrot, finely grated
½ tsp lemon juice
1 tsp ground cumin
2–3 tsp curry paste
⅓ cup all-purpose flour, plus extra for dusting
sunflower oil, for brushing
salt and pepper, to taste

1 Place the tofu, onion, carrot, lemon juice, cumin, and curry paste in a non-metallic bowl, combine well and marinate for at least an hour to allow the flavor of the spices to infuse the tofu.
2 Preheat the broiler to medium and line the broiler pan with foil. Stir in the flour until well mixed and season with salt and pepper. Shape the mixture into 10 cakes. Brush the cakes with oil and broil for 3 minutes. Turn them, brush with more oil, and cook for an additional 3 minutes until golden. Serve.

GARBANZO BEAN & EGGPLANT TAGINE

The sweetness of the dried apricots add to the popularity of this tasty vegetable and bean stew. Broiling the eggplant first helps to keep fat levels down, since eggplant is prone to absorbing a lot of oil when fried. Serve the tagine with plain couscous. Adults may like to add some chili!

Serves 4

1 tbsp olive oil, plus extra for brushing
1 large onion, chopped
1 carrot, diced
1 large eggplant, peeled and cut into bite-size pieces
1 red bell pepper, sliced
2 garlic cloves, chopped
1 tsp ground coriander
2 tsp ground cumin
1 tsp ground turmeric
2½ cups tomato purée
scant ½ cup vegetable bouillon
2 tsp tomato paste
10 ready-to-eat unsulfured apricots, chopped
¾ cup canned garbanzo beans, drained and rinsed
handful of pitted black olives (optional)
salt and pepper, to taste
1 tbsp chopped fresh cilantro, to garnish (optional)

1 Heat the olive oil in a large heavy-based saucepan over medium heat, add the onion and cook, covered, for 7 minutes until softened. Steam the carrot for 3 minutes until just tender.

2 Meanwhile, preheat the broiler to medium and line the broiler pan with foil. Arrange the eggplant pieces on the foil and brush with the extra oil. Broil for 6 minutes, turning the eggplant occasionally, or until browned and tender.

3 Add the bell pepper and garlic to the onion and cook, covered, stirring occasionally, for 2 minutes. Stir in the spices and cook for an additional minute.

4 Pour in the tomato purée and bouillon, stir in the tomato paste, and cook for 5 minutes, then add the apricots, garbanzo beans and olives, if using. Cook for 10 minutes, half-covered, stirring occasionally, or until reduced and thickened. Season to taste and serve with couscous. Sprinkle with fresh cilantro, if desired, just before serving.

BRAIN BOX

Vegetables, beans, and grains should play a major part in a healthy diet. For the brain, these slow-releasing carbohydrates provide sustained amounts of energy and aid concentration. Beans are also a good source of B-complex vitamins, iron, magnesium, and zinc.

REVITALIZING RICE

The combination of brown rice, lentils, eggs, and vegetables provides a powerful protein punch. This lightly spiced dish always goes down well with my family. It's good served in a chapati or soft tortilla.

B-complex vitamins, zinc, and iron are found in beneficial amounts in **lentils** and when combined with **brown rice and vegetables** form complementary proteins. This means that these ingredients when combined provide all the essential amino acids necessary to build neurotransmitters, the brain's vital messengers.

Serves 4–6

½ cup dried split red lentils
1 cup brown rice
1 tbsp olive oil
1 large onion, finely chopped
2 garlic cloves, crushed
1 tsp finely grated fresh gingerroot
½ tsp ground turmeric
2–3 tsp garam masala
2½ cups vegetable bouillon
1 carrot, diced
3 green beans, diagonally sliced
1 cup frozen peas
4 hard-boiled eggs, quartered
chapati or small soft tortilla, to serve (optional)

1 Rinse the lentils and rice separately under cold running water. Put the lentils in a pan and cover with cold water. Bring to a boil, then reduce the heat, skim off any foam that rises to the surface, and cook, half-covered, for 20 minutes or until tender. Drain well and set aside.

2 Meanwhile, heat the oil in a large heavy-based saucepan and cook the onion, covered, for 7 minutes until softened. Add the garlic and ginger and cook for an additional minute. Stir in the spices and rice and cook for another minute.

3 Add the vegetable bouillon to the rice and bring to a boil, then reduce the heat, cover, and simmer for 15 minutes. Add the carrot and green

beans, stir and cover again. Cook for an additional 20 minutes until the rice is tender and all the water has been absorbed, adding the peas 5 minutes before the end of the cooking time.

4 Gently stir the lentils into the spicy rice until combined. Spoon onto a chapati or tortilla, and top each serving with a hard-boiled egg. The chapati or tortilla can be rolled up, if preferred.

CLEVER CASHEW ROASTS

Cashews contain a whole range of brain-nourishing nutrients, so although nut roasts have become a bit of a vegetarian cliché, they offer significant health benefits. This version is very light and comes with a creamy onion sauce. Serve with roast potatoes, steamed broccoli, and brussels sprouts.

Serves 4
2 tbsp olive oil
2 onions, finely chopped
2 carrots, grated
1 parsnip, grated
2 tsp dried mixed herbs
1 tsp dried thyme
scant 1 cup unsalted cashew nuts
2 slices whole wheat bread, crusts removed
2 tbsp sunflower seeds
1 tbsp Worcestershire sauce (or vegetarian alternative)
1 tsp bouillon powder
2 eggs, beaten
salt and pepper, to taste

for the onion sauce:
large pat of butter
1 tsp olive oil
2 onions, finely chopped
1 tbsp all-purpose flour
1¼ cups milk, warmed
1 tsp Dijon mustard
good pinch of nutmeg
salt and pepper, to taste

1 To make the nut roast: preheat the oven to 400°F. Heat the oil in a large heavy-based saucepan, add the onion and cook, covered, for 7 minutes until softened. Add the carrots, parsnip, and herbs and cook for an additional 2 minutes. Remove the pan from the heat.
2 Meanwhile, grind the cashews in a food processor until finely chopped, then process the bread into crumbs. Stir into the pan with the seeds, Worcestershire sauce, and bouillon powder. Add the beaten eggs, season, and stir until combined.
3 Spoon the mixture into 4 individual greased dariole molds or 4-inch-diameter ring molds. Bake for 30 minutes until golden and crisp on top.
4 Meanwhile, make the onion sauce. Heat the butter and oil in a saucepan and cook the onions, covered, for 8 minutes until softened and beginning to brown. Add the flour, reduce the

heat, and stir continuously for 1 minute. Add half the warm milk and cook over medium-low heat, stirring, until it begins to thicken. Stir in the remaining milk and the mustard and cook for 6 minutes until it reaches a creamy consistency and there is no floury taste to the sauce. Season with the nutmeg and salt and pepper. Purée in a blender or food processor until smooth and creamy. Transfer to a pan and reheat if necessary.

TERIYAKI TUNA WITH NOODLES

Fresh tuna is part of the oily fish family and as such makes great brain food. It normally goes down well with children partly due to its firm, meaty texture and mild flavor. This dish comes with a light sesame noodle salad.

Serves 4
½ cup bottled teriyaki sauce
1 tsp honey
1lb fresh tuna, cut into strips
salt and pepper, to taste
1 tsp sesame seeds, to serve (optional)

for the noodle salad:
scant 2 cups uncooked medium egg noodles
3 tsp soy sauce
2 tsp sesame oil
1 tbsp olive oil
squeeze of lemon juice

BRAIN BOX

B-complex vitamins, omega-6 essential fatty acids, calcium, iron, magnesium, potassium, selenium, and zinc are among the multitude of brain-stimulating nutrients provided by **cashew nuts**. Cashews are, however, fairly high in fat and should be eaten in moderation.

½ tsp honey
4 tomatoes, de-seeded and chopped
2-in length of cucumber, diced
½ red bell pepper, de-seeded and diced
1 tbsp chopped fresh cilantro or basil
   (optional)
2 scallions, diagonally sliced

1 Combine the teriyaki sauce and honey and pour over the tuna. Turn the tuna in the marinade to coat it, season with salt and pepper, and leave it to marinate for at least 1 hour, turning the fish occasionally.

2 Meanwhile, to make the noodle salad, cook the noodles according to the package instructions. Drain well and rinse the noodles under cold running water. Mix together the soy sauce, sesame oil, olive oil, lemon juice, and honey and pour the dressing over the noodles. Add the tomatoes, cucumber, red bell pepper, cilantro or basil, if using, and scallions, and toss well to combine.

3 Heat a griddle pan or frying pan. Arrange the strips of tuna in the pan, pour over half the teriyaki sauce and cook for 2 minutes or until the fish is done to your taste, turning halfway and cooking in batches if necessary.

4 Spoon the noodle salad into four bowls and top with the strips of tuna. Sprinkle with sesame seeds, if desired.

MARVELOUS MEDITERRANEAN COD

This simple roasted cod and vegetable dish is served with a garlicky herb sauce, but if your children aren't into herbs, garlic mayonnaise works equally well. A salad is all that is needed as an accompaniment.

Serves 4
1¼ lb small new potatoes
2 tbsp olive oil
8 shallots, peeled
12 cherry tomatoes
3 sprigs fresh (½ tsp dried) oregano
4 thick-skinned cod fillets, about 1 lb
    5 oz total weight
1 lemon, sliced

for the herb sauce:
4 tbsp olive oil
1 garlic clove, crushed
4 tbsp chopped fresh parsley
2 tbsp chopped fresh mint
juice of ½ lemon
salt and pepper, to taste

1 Preheat the oven to 400°F. Wash and dry the potatoes and place them in a large roasting dish (you may need to use two) and toss in the oil. Roast in the oven for 30–35 minutes, turning occasionally. After 15 minutes, add the shallots and stir to coat with oil. Return to the oven.

2 Add the tomatoes and oregano to the vegetables and arrange the cod fillets on top. Season with salt and pepper. Top the fish with the lemon slices and bake for an additional 10 minutes or until the vegetables and potatoes are tender and the cod is cooked.
3 Meanwhile, put all the ingredients for the herb sauce in a blender and process until combined.
4 To serve, remove the herbs and lemon slices from the fish and arrange the potato-vegetable mixture, topped with fish, on four plates (children may prefer the fish cut into chunks). Accompany with the herb sauce.

BRAIN BOX

Fresh fish is a low-fat, high-protein source of B-complex vitamins, zinc, selenium, and calcium, vital for healthy nerves and mental processing.

CREAMY LENTIL & SMOKED HADDOCK CHOWDER

This comforting and sustaining thick soup is full of brain-stimulating goodness – make sure you buy naturally undyed smoked haddock, not the bright yellow variety. The soup makes a perfect weekend lunch served with crusty bread.

Serves 4
1¼ lb undyed smoked haddock fillets
milk, for poaching
1 cup dried split red lentils
1 bay leaf
1 large leek, sliced
1 carrot, sliced
1 stalk celery, sliced
3 cups vegetable bouillon
1¼ cups frozen corn kernels, thawed
    or 15½-oz can "no sugar or salt"
    corn kernels, drained and rinsed
2 tbsp sour cream or light cream
salt and pepper, to taste
1 tsp chopped chives or parsley, to serve

1 Place the smoked haddock in a large shallow pan and cover with milk. Poach for 8 minutes until cooked and opaque. Remove the fish from the pan, reserving the poaching liquid, and leave to cool. Remove the skin and any remaining bones and flake the fish into large pieces. Set aside.
2 Place the lentils, bay leaf, leek, carrot, celery, and bouillon in a large saucepan. Bring to a boil, skim off any

foam that rises to the surface, and reduce the heat. Simmer for 25–30 minutes, half-covered, until the lentils and vegetables are very tender, adding the corn 5 minutes before the end of the cooking time.

3 Remove the bay leaf and, using a hand blender or food processor, purée the soup slightly so that some vegetable pieces remain. Add ½ cup of the poaching milk and the sour cream or cream, stir well, and heat through. Gently mix in the fish, making sure you don't break up the chunks, and season to taste. Spoon into bowls and top with chopped chives or parsley.

STIMULATING SALMON CAKES WITH PEA PURÉE

Vegetable purées can be a useful way of encouraging children to eat their greens – here, the creamy pea sauce is flavored with mint. Fresh salmon is used but canned salmon makes a convenient alternative, albeit not as rich in omega-3 essential fatty acids.

Serves 4
¾ lb skinless salmon fillets
milk, for poaching
1½ lb potatoes, peeled and cut into
　　chunks
1 tbsp tomato ketchup
2 tsp Dijon mustard
2 scallions, thinly sliced
salt and pepper, to taste
flour, for dusting
sunflower oil, for frying

for the pea purée:
1 cup frozen peas
2 tbsp light cream
2 tsp chopped fresh mint
salt and pepper, to taste

1 Put the salmon in a large shallow pan and just cover with milk. Bring to a boil, then reduce the heat and simmer for 3–4 minutes until just cooked. Remove the fish from the pan and reserve the milk. Leave the salmon to cool slightly then flake the flesh into large chunks, removing any bones.

2 Meanwhile, boil the potatoes for 15 minutes or until very tender. Drain and mash with 2–3 tablespoons of the reserved poaching milk – you want quite dry yet lump-free mashed potatoes.

3 Stir the ketchup, mustard, scallions, and half of the salmon into the mashed potatoes. Season to taste. Mix thoroughly until well combined, then add the rest of the salmon to the potato mixture, mixing gently to avoid breaking up the fish.

4 Pour some flour onto a large plate. Lightly dust your hands with flour and shape the mixture into eight cakes. Dip each one in flour to coat lightly. Place the fish cakes on a baking sheet, cover with plastic wrap, and refrigerate for 30 minutes to firm up.

5 Heat enough oil to generously cover the base of a large frying pan. Cook the fish cakes, two or three at a time, for 3 minutes on each side until crisp and golden brown.

6 Meanwhile, cook the peas for 2 minutes. Drain well and transfer to a blender or food processor with the cream and mint. Purée, then season to taste. Reheat if necessary and serve with the fish cakes.

PERFECT IN PINK

Trout is another member of the oily fish family and its pale pink flesh has a light texture and mild fishy flavor. Here it is coated in a crispy milled oats coating and briefly pan-fried. You can find oatmeal in health food stores and some supermarkets. Serve the trout fillets with new potatoes and steamed vegetables.

Serves 4
4 trout fillets, about 1 lb total weight
medium oatmeal, for coating
salt and pepper, to taste
1 small egg, beaten
large pat of butter
2 tbsp sunflower oil, for frying
lemon wedges, for squeezing

for the sauce:
4 tbsp dill sauce
2 tbsp mayonnaise

1 Skin the fish using a small sharp knife, then rinse the fillets and pat dry with paper towels. Cut each one into 1-inch-wide strips.
2 Cover a plate with oatmeal and season it with salt and pepper. Dip each piece of fish in the beaten egg and then into the oats, until covered on both sides.
3 Heat half the butter and oil in a large heavy-based frying pan. Add half the trout strips and cook for 2 minutes on one side, turn over and cook for an additional minute; keep warm. Add the remaining butter and oil to the pan and cook the rest of the fish.
4 To make the sauce, mix together the dill sauce and mayonnaise. Divide the trout between four plates and serve with a spoonful of the sauce and a wedge of lemon for squeezing.

SPECIAL SHRIMP PASTA

This incredibly easy light pasta dish tastes special and is a perfect meal for the end of the day, when the pasta will help to calm the mind. Serve with a mixed salad.

Serves 4
½ lb whole wheat spaghetti
1 tbsp olive oil
1 large garlic clove, chopped
2 tsp dried oregano
¼ cup dry white wine
1⅔ cups tomato purée
½ tsp sugar
2 heaping tbsp cream cheese
¾ cup frozen peas, defrosted
6 oz cooked shrimp, defrosted if frozen
salt and pepper, to taste

1 Cook the pasta in plenty of boiling salted water according to the package instructions. Drain, reserving 2 tablespoons of the cooking water.
2 Meanwhile, heat the oil in a large heavy-based frying pan and cook the garlic and oregano for 1 minute until softened, taking care not to let the garlic burn. Add the wine and bring to a boil, then simmer over medium-high heat until the liquid has reduced slightly and no smell of alcohol remains.
3 Stir in the tomato purée and sugar, reduce the heat, and simmer for 10 minutes until reduced and thickened. Stir in the cream cheese, peas, and shrimp and season to taste. Cook for a few minutes until heated through.
4 Combine the pasta and reserved cooking water with the sauce and serve immediately.

BRAIN BOX

Shrimp is a good source of zinc, which is needed by the pituitary gland. A lack of zinc can lead to mood swings, irritability, and depression.

ROASTED RED PESTO CHICKEN

Chicken is an excellent source of low-fat protein, but make sure you buy organic, free-range poultry for improved flavor and quality. This dish includes a recipe for red pesto but you can use a ready-made version, if preferred, opting for a good-quality one. Serve with roast potatoes and plenty of veggies.

Serves 4
4 skinless, boneless chicken breasts, about 1¼ lb total weight
1 tbsp olive oil
2 tbsp pine nuts

for the red pesto:
½ cup sun-dried tomatoes in oil, drained and chopped
2 garlic cloves, crushed
4 tbsp pine nuts
⅔ cup extra-virgin olive oil
¾ cup freshly grated Parmesan cheese

1 Preheat the oven to 400°F. To make the red pesto, put the ingredients in a food processor and blend until they form a coarse purée.
2 Arrange the chicken in a large ovenproof dish. Brush each breast with the oil then spread a tablespoon of red pesto over each one until completely covered. Any leftover pesto can be stored in an airtight container in the refrigerator for up to a week.
3 Roast the chicken for 30 minutes or until the juices run clear when it is pierced with a skewer and there is no sign of any pink.
4 Meanwhile, lightly toast the pine nuts in a dry frying pan. Arrange the chicken breasts on four plates and sprinkle with the nuts and serve with roast potatoes and steamed vegetables.

BRAIN BOX

Selenium, zinc, and B-complex vitamins, all of which are essential to brain function, are found in **turkey**. **Shrimp** is also a good source of zinc, while the **peas** provide plentiful amounts of vitamin C and beta-carotene.

PEACEFUL PAELLA

Experts have found that rice contains tryptophan, which helps to boost the production of the calming chemical serotonin. Turkey has a similar effect, so a good night's sleep is in the cards!

Serves 4
2 tbsp olive oil
1 large onion, diced
2 skinless, boneless turkey breasts, about ¾ lb total weight, cut into bite-size pieces
1 red bell pepper, de-seeded and diced
2 garlic cloves, chopped
2 tomatoes, de-seeded and chopped
1 tbsp tomato paste
pinch of saffron
3½ cups hot chicken or vegetable bouillon
generous 1 cup paella rice
1 cup frozen peas
generous ½ cup cooked shrimp, defrosted if frozen
salt and pepper, to taste

1 Heat the oil in a large heavy-based lidded sauté pan. Add the onion and cook, covered, for 7 minutes or until softened. Add the turkey, red bell pepper, and garlic and cook for 5 minutes over medium heat, stirring frequently, until the turkey is browned all over.
2 Add the tomato, tomato paste, saffron, and bouillon to the pan. Stir in the rice and bring to a boil. Reduce the heat and simmer, covered, for 15–20 minutes or until the rice is tender.
3 Add the peas, shrimp, and seasoning and cook for an additional 2 minutes, stirring frequently, until the shrimp has heated through and the peas are cooked. Serve immediately.

TIME-FOR-BED FRICASSEE

This creamy yet low-fat dish features a healthy combination of turkey, vegetables, and beans. Served with rice, it makes a balanced and brain-nourishing light supper. The white wine adds a rounded flavor to the dish and as the alcohol is cooked out, there are none of the negative effects – but you can leave it out and increase the amount of bouillon accordingly.

Serves 4

1 tbsp all-purpose flour
salt and pepper, to taste
4 skinless turkey breasts, about 1¼ lb total weight, cut into bite-size pieces
1 tbsp olive oil
1 large onion, finely chopped
2 garlic cloves, chopped
1 red bell pepper, de-seeded and diced
2 tsp dried oregano
2 carrots, finely diced
2 ears fresh corn, shucked, kernels scraped off
¼ cup dry white wine
⅔ cup chicken or vegetable bouillon
4 tbsp reduced-fat sour cream
¾ cup canned flageolet or navy beans, drained and rinsed

1 Sprinkle the flour on a plate and season with salt and pepper. Toss the turkey pieces in the flour. Heat the oil in a large heavy-based lidded sauté pan over medium heat and fry the onion for 7 minutes. Remove the onion and add the turkey pieces. Brown for 5–10 minutes, turning the meat often to prevent it burning. Add a little stock to the pan if the meat begins to stick.
2 Return the onion to the pan with the garlic, bell pepper, and oregano and cook for an additional 2–3 minutes until the pepper has softened. Add the carrots, corn kernels, and white wine, then increase the heat and boil until the liquid has reduced and the alcohol has evaporated – any smell of wine should have disappeared.
3 Reduce the heat, add the bouillon, and cook, covered, for 10 minutes. Stir in the sour cream and beans and heat through. Season to taste and serve.

> **BRAIN** BOX
>
> Make sure you use good-quality lean **organic pork** for this recipe. Red meat is a good source of iron, a lack of which is common in children and has been linked to behavioral problems, including mood swings, irritability, and hyperactivity.

PORK & APPLE PAN-FRY

Pork tenderloin is used here because it is lean and cooks quickly. The apple is perfect with pork and the beans add healthy low-fat protein and vital brain minerals. Serve with new potatoes or rice and salad.

Serves 4

1 tbsp all-purpose flour
1 tsp paprika
1½ lb pork tenderloin, trimmed and cut into bite-size pieces
1½ tbsp olive oil
1 large onion, finely chopped
1 large eating apple, pared, cored, and cut into bite-size pieces
1 tbsp chopped fresh rosemary
1¼ cups vegetable bouillon
2 tomatoes, de-seeded and roughly chopped
1½ cups canned flageolet or navy beans, drained and rinsed
2 tbsp low-fat sour cream
salt and pepper, to taste

1 Mix together the flour and paprika on a plate. Add the pork pieces and toss in the seasoned flour, shaking off any excess flour.

2 Heat the oil in a heavy-based frying pan over medium heat, add the pork and cook for 5 minutes, turning the meat until browned all over. Add the onion and cook for an additional 7 minutes until softened. Mix in the apple and rosemary and cook for 3–4 minutes until the apples begin to break up.

3 Pour in the bouillon, bring to a boil, reduce the heat, and simmer for 15 minutes until reduced and thickened. Stir in the tomatoes and beans, then cook for an additional 10 minutes over low heat. Stir in the sour cream and heat through. Season to taste and serve.

COTTAGE PIE WITH A TWIST

I've used ground beef here but this mildly spiced cottage pie can be made with a vegetarian alternative if preferred. Add the meat substitute at step 4, with the spices. Steamed broccoli and snow peas are perfect accompaniments.

Serves 4
1½ tbsp olive oil
1 onion, finely chopped
1 lb lean ground beef
1 carrot, grated
1 stalk celery, finely chopped
2 garlic cloves, chopped
1 bay leaf
¼ cup dry white wine (optional)
1 tsp paprika
1 tsp ground cumin
1 tsp ground coriander
2½ cups tomato purée
⅔ cup vegetable bouillon
¾ cup canned cannellini beans,
   drained and rinsed
salt and pepper, to taste
2 tsp sesame seeds

for the mashed sweet potatoes:
½ lb sweet potatoes, peeled and cut
   into chunks
1 lb potatoes, peeled and cut into
   chunks
2 tbsp butter
½ cup warm milk

1 Preheat the oven to 400°F. To make the mashed sweet potatoes, cook both types of potato in boiling salted water for 15 minutes until tender. Drain and add the butter and warm milk. Mash until smooth and season to taste; set aside.

2 Meanwhile, heat the oil in a large heavy-based saucepan and cook the onion, covered, for 7 minutes until softened. Stir in the meat and cook, stirring frequently, until browned. Add the carrot, celery, garlic, and bay leaf and cook, covered, for another 5 minutes, stirring frequently.

3 Add the wine, increase the heat, and boil for 3 minutes until reduced and the alcohol has evaporated. Add the spices and cook for 1 minute, stirring frequently, then pour in the tomato purée and bouillon. Bring to a boil, reduce the heat, and stir in the beans. Simmer, half-covered, for 10 minutes until reduced and thickened and season to taste.

4 Transfer the meat mixture to an ovenproof dish and spoon the mashed potatoes over. Spread the mash with the back of a spoon until the meat is covered, then sprinkle the top with sesame seeds. Bake for 25–30 minutes until the mashed potatoes begin to crisp and brown on top.

SAUSAGE & BEAN HOTPOT

Good-quality pork sausages are used in this warming, substantial stew, but you could quite easily use vegetarian ones. Beans, vegetables, and nuts are also included to provide a wide range of brain-boosting nutrients. Serve with a baked potato and a green vegetable.

Serves 4

8 good-quality pork or vegetarian
   sausages
2 tbsp olive oil
1 large onion, finely chopped
2 garlic cloves, chopped
1 tsp dried thyme
1 tsp dried mixed herbs
1 red bell pepper, de-seeded and diced
1½ lb butternut squash, de-seeded,
   peeled and cut into bite-size pieces
¾ cup fresh apple juice
1½ cups vegetable or chicken bouillon
1 tsp Dijon mustard
¾ cup canned cannellini beans,
   drained and rinsed
2 heaping tbsp unsalted, raw
   cashew nuts
¼ cup milk
1 slice whole wheat bread, crusts
   removed and broken into pieces
salt and pepper, to taste

BRAIN BOX

Butternut squash contains antioxidants beta-carotene, lycopene, and vitamin C, which help to promote mental alertness and memory by protecting nerve cells in the brain. **Red bell peppers** have similar properties.

1 Preheat the broiler to medium-high and line a broiler pan with foil. Broil the sausages, turning occasionally, until browned and cooked through. Set aside.
2 Meanwhile, heat the oil in a large saucepan over medium heat. Add the onion and fry, covered, for about 7 minutes, stirring occasionally, until softened. Add the garlic, herbs, and bell pepper and cook, covered, for an additional 3 minutes. Stir in the butternut squash, stir well, and cook for 5 minutes.

3 Pour in the apple juice. Increase the heat, bring to a boil, and cook for 3 minutes until the juice has reduced. Lower the heat to medium, pour in the bouillon, stir in the mustard and beans and cook, uncovered, for 15 minutes.
4 While the hotpot is cooking, grind the nuts in a food processor, then add the milk and bread. Continue to process to make a thick paste. Stir the paste into the hotpot – this will help to thicken the liquid. Cook for another 5 minutes until thickened and season to taste before serving.

BRAIN BOX

Lean **organic beef** can play a part in a healthy diet if eaten in moderation. Meat is a complete protein and a good source of iron, zinc, and some B-complex vitamins in a readily absorbable form. A lack of iron has been linked to learning difficulties and poor concentration. Organic beef is free from the cocktail of chemicals such as hormones and growth promoters that intensively reared animals are often exposed to.

AUTUMN BEEFY BRAINY STEW

It is important to use good-quality organic beef for this hearty stew. Don't be put off by the length of time it takes to cook, since it doesn't require any lengthy involvement from the cook and the slow-cooking results in a rich, thick gravy and succulent meat. Serve with mashed potatoes and a green vegetable.

Serves 4

3 tbsp all-purpose flour
salt and pepper, to taste
1½ lb lean diced organic casserole beef
3 tbsp olive oil
12 shallots, peeled and halved or
　 quartered if large
2 carrots, cut into batons
1 parsnip, sliced into circles
2 bay leaves
1 tbsp chopped fresh rosemary
1 tbsp chopped fresh thyme
1¾ cups brown ale
1 cup beef bouillon
1 tbsp Worcestershire sauce
18 canned chestnuts,
　 drained

1 Preheat the oven to 325°F. Put the flour in a clean plastic food bag or on a plate and season generously. Toss the beef in the seasoned flour until coated. Heat 1 tbsp oil in a large flameproof, ovenproof casserole dish. Add one-third of the beef and cook for 5–6 minutes, turning occasionally, until browned all over – the meat may stick to the pan until it is properly sealed. Remove the browned beef from the pan and cook the remaining two batches, adding another 1 tbsp oil when necessary. Set aside when all the beef has been sealed.

2 Add the remaining oil to the pan with the shallots, carrots, parsnip, and herbs and cook for 3 minutes, stirring occasionally.

3 Pour in the ale and bring to a boil. Cook over a high heat until the alcohol in the ale has evaporated and the liquid has reduced. Add the bouillon and Worcestershire sauce, then cook for another 3 minutes.

4 Stir in the chestnuts and beef. Make sure the liquid returns to a boil, then cover the dish and transfer to the oven. Cook for 2 hours until the stock has formed a rich gravy and the meat is tender. Season to taste before serving.

PICNICS AND PARTIES

Finding a good range of nutritious picnic and party food can be quite a challenge, but this section contains a selection of innovative and fun sweet and savory recipes that will appeal to everyone.

MAGIC FAIRY BOWL

If your kids need extra encouragement to eat fruit, this pretty party piece may be just the thing. The hollowed out melon is filled with fruit of your choice to give a stunning result.

Serves 6
½ large Charentais, cantaloupe, or
　honeydew melon, seeds scooped out
a selection of fruits, such as
　strawberries, raspberries, slices of
　nectarine or peach, orange sections,
　or seedless grapes

1 Cut a sliver off the base of the melon so it stands upright and place on a serving plate. Scoop out most of the flesh using a melon baller or teaspoon to leave a hollow bowl shape, setting the fruit aside.
2 Fill the melon half with the fruit of your choice mixed with the melon balls, pouring over any juice.

BRAIN BOX

Melons, particularly the orange-fleshed variety, contain useful amounts of the brain-protecting antioxidants beta-carotene and vitamin C as well as folic acid and vitamin B_6.

MELON BOATS

Fun and healthy, too, these melon sailing boats are a simple idea but make a great addition to any party. Choose natural cheese slices to avoid unwanted additives. Take care when offering these boats to very small children because of the cocktail sticks.

Makes 12 boats
1 small melon, such as galia,
　Charentais, or cantaloupe
12 natural cheese slices, like Gruyère,
　Edam, or Cheddar
12 cocktail sticks (toothpicks)

1 Cut the melon in half and scoop out the seeds. Cut each half into 6 wedges.
2 Thread each cheese slice onto a cocktail stick so that the slices look like sails with the sticks for the masts. You could fix a paper flag on the top of each stick.
3 Place each cheese sail into a melon wedge to make the boats and serve.

HALLOUMI, HAM, & PINEAPPLE STICKS

Children love these, but take care when serving them to young children. Halloumi cheese – great for cooking because it retains its shape – is available from Greek delis and speciality stores. If possible, use fresh instead of canned pineapple, since it is richer in vitamins. Cherry tomatoes, bacon, and nectarine slices make tasty alternatives.

BRAIN BOX

Pineapple contains manganese, which aids poor memory by improving oxygenation and protecting brain tissue.

Makes 12 sticks
½ lb halloumi cheese, cut into
　24 cubes
1 small pineapple, peeled and cored
2 thick slices good-quality lean ham,
　cut into 24 cubes
12 cocktail sticks (toothpicks)

1 Preheat the broiler to high and line the broiler pan with foil. Arrange the cubes of halloumi in the pan and broil lightly, turning occasionally, until just golden. Leave to cool slightly.
2 Cut the pineapple into thick slices and cut into 24 chunks.
3 Thread a chunk of pineapple onto a cocktail stick, followed by a cube of halloumi and a cube of ham. Repeat to make 12 sticks.

PIZZA PRESTO!

By making your own pizzas you can avoid the unwanted additives often included in overprocessed store-bought versions. This pizza is perfect when time is short, since the base doesn't require prolonged kneading and rising.

Makes 8
½ cup whole wheat flour
1½ cups all-purpose flour
1 tbsp baking powder
2 tsp dried oregano
1 tsp salt
4 tbsp olive oil

for the topping:
1 tbsp olive oil
1 garlic clove, crushed
1¼ cups tomato purée
2 tsp sun-dried tomato paste
8 slices mozzarella cheese
2 tbsp grated Cheddar cheese

1 To make the pizza bases, combine the two different types of flour, baking powder, oregano, and salt in a mixing bowl. Add 2 tablespoons of the olive oil and 5 fl oz water. Mix with your hands to make a soft dough.

2 Turn out the dough on a lightly floured work surface. Knead until it forms a smooth dough then wrap in plastic wrap and allow to rest while you make the tomato sauce.

3 To make the tomato sauce, heat the olive oil in a medium-size heavy-based saucepan over medium-low heat. Fry the garlic for 1 minute then add the tomato purée and tomato paste and cook for 8 minutes, stirring occasionally, until reduced and thickened.

4 Meanwhile, divide the dough into 8 pieces and roll out each piece into a circle, about 2½ inches in diameter. Heat half the remaining oil in a large heavy-based frying pan. Arrange half of the pizza bases in the pan and cook for 2–3 minutes on each side until golden. Keep warm while you cook the remaining pizza bases, adding the rest of the oil if necessary.

5 Preheat the broiler to medium-high. Spread the tomato sauce over the bases and top each one with a slice of mozzarella and a sprinkling of Cheddar. Broil for 1–2 minutes until the mozzarella has melted and is beginning to turn golden.

BRAIN BOX

B-complex vitamins provided by **eggs and ham** help feed the brain to improve mental clarity and motivation.

PICNIC PIES

There's no high-fat pastry in these pies; instead a slice of good-quality lean ham is used as a base for the quiche-style filling. They are just as delicious cold as warm and are the right size for children to hold.

Makes 8
butter, for greasing
8 small slices lean good-quality ham
3 eggs, beaten
1 cup milk
scant ½ cup grated sharp Cheddar cheese
freshly ground pepper
2 tomatoes, sliced

1 Preheat the oven to 350°F. Lightly grease an 8-hole muffin pan with some butter. Line the base and sides of each pan with a slice of ham, folding the ham where necessary, to make cup shapes.

2 Mix together the eggs, milk, and cheese, season with a little pepper, and pour the mixture into each ham-lined muffin pan. Top each one with a slice of tomato and bake for 15–20 minutes until the egg filling has risen and set. Leave to cool slightly then transfer to a wire rack to cool further. Serve warm or cold.

HAPPY CHICKEN STICKS

Chicken is a high-quality, low-fat – as long as the skin has been removed – protein, but make sure you buy organic, free-range meat to avoid added chemicals. Try these dipped into satay sauce (see page 70).

Makes 16
4 skinless, boneless chicken breasts, about 1 lb total weight
2 tbsp olive oil
juice of ½ lemon
salt and freshly ground pepper, to taste

1 Soak 16 wooden skewers in a bowl of water for 30 minutes to prevent them from burning. Cut each chicken breast lengthwise into four strips and thread each one onto a skewer.
2 Combine the olive oil, lemon juice, and seasoning in a small bowl then brush the chicken with the mixture.
3 Heat a griddle pan to medium-hot. Cook the chicken skewers for 3 minutes on each side until golden and cooked through, making sure there is no trace of pink inside. Cook for slightly longer if there is any sign of pinkness.

TUNA & LEEK FRITTATA

Transported whole or cut into chunky wedges, a frittata makes a protein-rich nutritious addition to a picnic or packed lunch box that will fight hunger pangs and provide plenty of brain energy for the rest of the day.

Serves 4–6
1 tbsp olive oil
small pat of butter
1 large leek, finely sliced
7-oz can tuna in olive oil or spring water, drained
6 eggs, beaten
salt and pepper, to taste

1 Heat the oil and butter in a medium-size flameproof frying pan then fry the leek for 5–7 minutes until softened. Stir in the tuna, making sure that there is an even distribution of leek and tuna and that some chunks of tuna remain.
2 Preheat the broiler to medium-high. Season the beaten eggs and pour them carefully over the tuna and leek mixture. Cook over moderate heat for 5 minutes or until the eggs are just set and the base of the frittata is golden brown.
3 Place the pan under the broiler and cook the top of the frittata for 3 minutes or until set and lightly golden. Serve the frittata warm or cold, cut into wedges or fingers.

FIRED-UP FALAFEL

Beans, with the exception of the baked variety, are often neglected in children's diets, but they offer a beneficial range of vital minerals for the brain. Serve these falafel in mini sesame-seed-coated pita breads along with some hummus and salad leaves of your choice – yum!

Makes 12 falafel
14-oz can garbanzo beans, drained
    and rinsed
2 cloves garlic, crushed
2 scallions, finely sliced
1 tsp ground cumin
1 tsp ground coriander
1 tbsp sesame seeds
1 egg, beaten
flour, for dusting
sunflower oil, for frying
mini sesame-seed pita breads, red
    pepper hummus (see page 59) and
    salad leaves, to serve

1 Put the garbanzo beans, garlic, scallions, cumin, coriander, and sesame seeds in a food processor and blend until the beans are roughly chopped. Add the egg and blend again until the mixture forms a coarse paste. Place in the refrigerator for 1 hour to allow the mixture to firm up.

2 Form the mixture into 12 walnut-size balls using lightly floured hands, then roll in flour until lightly coated.

BRAIN BOX

Beans are a useful blend of protein and carbohydrate and are low in fat to boot. These nutrients work in tandem to build the brain's neurotransmitters and provide long-term energy.

3 Heat 1 tablespoon oil in a large heavy-based frying pan and cook the falafel in batches (adding more oil if necessary) for 6 minutes, turning occasionally, until golden. Drain on paper towels.
4 Warm each pita bread and split along one side. Spread the inside with hummus and place two falafel in each one (you could cut them in half if easier to handle). Add the salad leaves of your choice and serve.

BETTER-FOR-YOU BABY BURGERS

By using good-quality, preferably organic, ingredients, you can have a healthy and delicious burger in next to no time.

Makes 10 burgers
¾ cup fresh whole wheat bread
    crumbs
1 tsp dried oregano
1 onion, grated
1 carrot, finely grated

1 garlic clove, crushed
1 lb lean ground beef or vegetarian
   alternative
1 egg, beaten
salt and pepper, to taste
flour, for dusting
sunflower oil, for frying
10 whole wheat mini burger buns,
   to serve
sliced tomato and lettuce leaves,
   to serve
mayonnaise, relish, or tomato ketchup,
   to serve (optional)

1 Place the bread crumbs, oregano, onion, carrot, garlic, beef, and egg in a large bowl. Season and mix with your hands until all the ingredients are combined. Shape the mixture into 10 smallish balls using floured hands. Set aside in the refrigerator for 15 minutes.
2 Heat enough oil to lightly cover the bottom of a large heavy-based frying pan. Place the balls in the hot oil, flattening each one with a spatula, and fry in batches for 3 minutes on each side until browned and cooked through.
3 Split the burger buns in half and add the burgers. Serve with sliced tomato, lettuce, and the accompaniment of your choice.

PICNIC FOCACCIA

There's something very satisfying about making bread, and children love to get involved in the kneading and shaping.

Serves 6–8
2¼ cups whole wheat bread flour
2¼ cups white bread flour, plus extra
   for dusting
¼ oz package instant dried yeast
2 tsp salt
1⅓ cups lukewarm water
½ lb mozzarella cheese, sliced
handful fresh basil leaves
8 sun-dried tomatoes, roughly sliced
1 tsp oil from the tomatoes or extra-
   virgin olive oil
2 tsp extra-virgin olive oil
coarse sea salt, for sprinkling (optional)

1 Combine both types of flour with the yeast and salt in a large mixing bowl. Make a well in the center and pour in the water. Stir initially with a wooden spoon and then with your hands. Knead to make a soft, slightly sticky dough, adding a little more water or flour if the dough is too dry or wet.
2 Turn out the dough on a lightly floured work surface. Knead for 10 minutes – push the dough flat with the palm of your hand, fold the far edge toward you, giving it a half turn, then repeat the process. Place the dough in the clean bowl, cover with a kitchen towel and leave it to rest somewhere warm and out of a draft

for 45–60 minutes until doubled in size.
3 Divide the dough into two pieces. Roll out each piece into an 8½-inch circle and place one circle on a lightly floured baking sheet. Top with the cheese, basil leaves, and tomatoes. Sprinkle the oil from the tomatoes over the top.
4 Place the other circle of dough on top, pressing down the edges firmly over the filling to seal. Cover the focaccia with a kitchen towel and set aside for another 30 minutes to rise. Preheat the oven to 425°F.
5 Make indentations in the bread with your fingers, sprinkle the olive oil over the top and the coarse sea salt, if using. Bake for 35 minutes until risen and golden. Remove from the baking sheet and tap the base of the bread with your fingers – it should sound hollow when done. Leave to cool on a wire rack.

BRAIN BOX

Protein supplied by the **cheese** and carbohydrates in the **flour** work together to keep blood glucose levels steady and consequently help to avoid dips in concentration and mental alertness.

SUPER SEEDY BREAD STICKS

Children will love making these bread sticks, which make healthy energy-boosting snacks eaten on their own or dipped into hummus or similar alternative. Store in an airtight container for a couple of days or freeze for later use.

Makes about 55 bread sticks
4 tbsp sunflower seeds
3 tbsp olive oil
2¼ cups white bread flour, plus extra for dusting
2¼ cups whole wheat bread flour
¼ oz package instant dried yeast
1½ tsp salt
1¼ cups lukewarm water
1 egg, beaten
1 tbsp milk
sesame seeds, for sprinkling

1 Lightly toast the sunflower seeds in a dry frying pan. Transfer to a food processor with 1 tablespoon of the olive oil and grind to make a rough paste. Set aside to cool.
2 Combine both types of flour with the yeast and salt. Add the ground seeds, water, and the rest of the oil, mixing initially with a wooden spoon and then your hands to make a soft, slightly sticky dough, adding more water or flour if the dough seems too dry or wet.

3 Dust the work surface with flour and knead the dough for 10 minutes – push it flat with the palm of your hand, then fold the far edge toward you, giving it a half turn, then repeat the process. Place the dough in a clean bowl, cover with a kitchen towel and leave it to rest somewhere warm and out of a draft for 10 minutes.
4 Preheat the oven to 425°F. Roll out the dough into a very thin rectangle, halve the dough horizontally and cut into ½ inch-wide strips. Roll each piece of dough into a sausage-shape using both hands and place on lightly floured

BRAIN BOX

Calcium, zinc, magnesium, potassium, vitamin E, and omega-6 essential fatty acids (EFAs) are found in beneficial amounts in **sunflower seeds**. EFAs are crucial for healthy brain development and have to be supplied by diet since the body is not able to make them itself.

baking sheets. You will probably need about 3 baking sheets, as this dough makes about 55 bread sticks. Cover each sheet with a clean kitchen towel and set aside for 15 minutes until risen.
5 Mix together the beaten egg and milk and brush over each bread stick. Sprinkle each one with sesame seeds and bake for 15 minutes until crisp and golden. Transfer to a wire rack to cool.

FRUITY SODA BREAD

Soda bread is the perfect introduction to bread making for children – it doesn't require lengthy kneading or rising as it doesn't contain yeast. Although dried fruit is high in natural sugars, it does provide valuable minerals that work synergistically to boost mental performance.

Serves 6–8
2 cups white bread flour, plus extra for dusting
2 cups whole wheat bread flour
1½ tsp salt
1 tsp baking powder
1 heaping tbsp superfine sugar
1 cup ready-to-eat pitted prunes or dates, roughly chopped
1 egg, lightly beaten
1¼ cups buttermilk
2–3 tbsp yogurt with live and active cultures or milk (optional)

1 Preheat the oven to 400°F. Sift together both types of flour with the salt and baking soda into a large bowl, adding any bran left in the sieve. Add the sugar and prunes and mix well to combine.

2 Make a well in the center of the mixture and add the beaten egg and buttermilk. Mix initially with a wooden spoon and then your hands to form a soft, slightly sticky dough. If the dough is too dry, add the yogurt or milk.

3 Turn out the dough on a lightly floured work surface and knead lightly until the dough is smooth. Form into a flat circle, about 1½ inches thick.

4 Place the loaf on a floured baking sheet and dust with flour. Cut a large deep cross in the dough then bake for 30–35 minutes until risen and golden – the bread should sound hollow when tapped on the bottom with your fingers. Transfer to a wire rack to cool.

BRAIN BOX

Whole wheat flour is richer in B-complex vitamins, fiber, vitamin E, selenium, and magnesium than its refined white counterpart. A lack of B-complex vitamins can affect mental judgment and increase anxiety.

PARTY PEOPLE

These mini "people-shaped" cheese biscuits make a fun addition to a party table without containing heaps of sugar. Spread with cream cheese for a protein boost.

Makes 12 people
1 cup all-purpose flour, plus extra for dusting
1 cup whole wheat flour
2 tsp baking powder
large pinch of salt
4 tbsp chilled butter, cubed
3 tbsp freshly grated Parmesan cheese
1 egg, beaten
scant ½ cup milk, plus extra for glazing

1 Preheat the oven to 425°F and lightly grease 2 baking sheets. Sift both types of flour with the baking powder into a large bowl, and mix in the salt.

2 Rub in the butter with your fingertips until the mixture forms coarse bread crumbs. Stir in the cheese. Make a well in the center of the mixture and pour in the egg and milk. Mix initially with a wooden spoon and then with your hands to make a soft dough.

3 Turn out the dough on a lightly floured work surface and gently press into a circle about 1 inch thick. Stamp out 12 biscuits using a small gingerbread man/woman cutter. Place on the prepared baking sheets, brush the tops with milk, and bake for 15 minutes, until risen and golden. Transfer to a wire rack to cool.

CARROT CAKE

This recipe makes a sizeable two-layer birthday cake but it can be halved for an everyday cake. What's more, your children will never guess that this light, moist cake contains healthy carrots!

Serves 20
butter, for greasing
4 cups all-purpose flour
2 tsp baking powder
1 tsp salt
2 tsp ground cinnamon
2 tsp ground nutmeg
2 cups light brown sugar
1 lb carrots, grated
6 eggs, beaten
scant 1½ cups sunflower oil

for the frosting:
scant ¾ cup cream cheese
6 tbsp unsalted butter
1 tsp natural vanilla extract
¾ cup unrefined powdered sugar

to decorate:
low-sugar, natural-fruit gumdrops,
chocolate sprinkles, candles

1 Preheat the oven to 350°F. Lightly grease two 8-inch-square or 9-inch-round cake pans with butter and line the bases with parchment paper.
2 Sift the flour, baking powder, salt, and spices into a large mixing bowl. Add the sugar and carrots and mix well.

3 Mix together the eggs and oil then add to the mixture in the bowl, stirring with a wooden spoon until combined.
4 Pour the mixture into the prepared cake pans, level with the back of a spoon, and bake for 40 minutes or until a toothpick inserted into the center of each cake comes out clean. Leave for 10 minutes, then carefully turn out the cakes to cool on wire racks.
5 To make the frosting, beat together the cream cheese, butter, and vanilla extract until light and creamy. Beat in the powdered sugar, then place in the refrigerator for 15 minutes to harden slightly.
6 Level off the top of each cake with a knife then spread the frosting over one cake. Place the second cake on top and spread with a final layer of frosting – it doesn't matter if it runs down the sides. Decorate with the gumdrops and chocolate sprinkles. Candles add the finishing touch for a birthday or other celebration.

VARIATION
Swap the carrots for 6 mashed ripe bananas; the combination of bananas and nutmeg are said to encourage restful sleep.

NUTTY COLESLAW

This is nothing like commercially made coleslaws, where the artificial-tasting vegetables are dripping in dressing with a smattering of the usual preservatives and other additives. For the optimum amount of nutrients and best flavor, prepare this version as close to serving as possible.

BRAIN BOX

Cabbage and carrots are rich in antioxidants and help to protect the brain from damaging toxins.

Pumpkin seeds are one of the few foods to contain both omega-3 and omega-6 essential fatty acids.

Walnuts and olive oil further boost the essential fatty acid content, which are vital for an efficient nervous system and healthy brain cells.

Serves 6
1 heaping cup finely shredded white cabbage
2 carrots, grated
2 scallions, finely sliced on the diagonal
1 tbsp chopped walnuts (or other nuts of your choice)
2 tbsp pumpkin or sunflower seeds
1 eating apple, pared, cored, and diced

for the dressing:
2 tbsp extra-virgin olive oil
1 tbsp fresh lemon juice, plus extra for coating
4 tbsp mayonnaise

1 Mix together the cabbage, carrots, and scallions in a salad bowl. Lightly toast the nuts and seeds in a dry frying pan for 2 minutes. Leave to cool. Stir the cooled nuts and seeds into the salad.
2 Mix together the ingredients for the dressing and pour it over the salad. Toss well to coat. Toss the apple pieces in the extra lemon juice to prevent them from browning and sprinkle the apple over the top of the salad before serving.

BRAIN BOX

Couscous as a carbohydrate has a soothing, calming effect on the brain. Similarly, **basil**, which is found in the pesto, is a calming and mood-enhancing herb.

The protein in the **halloumi cheese**, however, will help to stimulate and enliven the mind.

CALMING COUSCOUS

If you can't find halloumi cheese, substitute cubed feta cheese and add it – uncooked – to the couscous.

Serves 4
scant 2 cups uncooked couscous
½ cup cubed halloumi cheese
2–3 tbsp green or red pesto, to taste
2 tsp olive oil
10 cherry tomatoes, halved

1 Preheat the broiler to medium and line the broiler pan with foil. Put the couscous into a bowl, then pour over boiling water to cover by a ¼ inch. Stir, then set aside until the water has been absorbed by the couscous. Fluff up with a fork and taste – if the couscous is still hard, add a little more boiling water and leave for a few minutes more.
2 Arrange the halloumi cheese in the broiler pan and broil for a few minutes, turning occasionally, until golden.

3 Stir the pesto and oil into the couscous until it is thoroughly coated. Mix in the tomatoes and broiled halloumi and serve.

CARAMEL SESAME POPCORN

Good fun and incredibly easy to cook, popcorn is a party must. Additionally, this version is much lower in sugar than store-bought popcorn and is also free of additives.

Serves 6–8
sunflower oil
½ cup popping corn
2 tbsp unsalted butter
3 tbsp maple syrup
2 tbsp sesame seeds

1 Heat enough oil (about 1 tablespoon) to cover the bottom of a medium-size, heavy-based, lidded saucepan. When hot, add the popping corn in a single layer and cover with the lid. Cook over medium heat, shaking the pan frequently, until the corn has popped. Do not lift the lid until the corn has finished popping. Transfer the popcorn to a large bowl.
2 Melt the butter in the pan and add the maple syrup. Bring to a boil then reduce the heat and simmer briefly until thickened. Leave to cool slightly, then pour the buttery maple syrup over the popcorn and add the sesame seeds. Toss well to thoroughly coat the popcorn in the mixture. Leave to cool before serving.

BRAIN BOX

Corn is one of the most nutritionally balanced carbohydrates and as such is a good food for the brain and nervous system.

FEEL-GOOD BROWNIES

Chocolate boosts endorphin and serotonin levels in the brain, having an uplifting effect and encouraging a buoyant mood. That said, it should be eaten in moderation, since chocolate also contains the stimulants caffeine and theobromine.

Makes 24 brownies

2 sticks unsalted butter, plus extra
    for greasing
7 oz good-quality bittersweet
    chocolate (at least 50 percent
    cocoa solids)
¾ cup roughly chopped hazelnuts
3 eggs, beaten
1 cup unrefined superfine sugar
1½ cups all-purpose flour
1 tsp baking powder
½ cup chopped ready-to-eat
    pitted dates

1 Preheat the oven to 350°F. Grease a 12 x 8-inch baking pan with the extra butter and line with parchment paper.
2 Break up the chocolate and place it with the butter in a heatproof bowl. Place the bowl over a pan of barely simmering water and heat until the chocolate and butter have melted, stirring once or twice. Set aside to cool slightly.
3 Meanwhile, lightly toast the hazelnuts in a dry frying pan until beginning to turn golden brown. Set aside to cool.

BRAIN BOX

These brownies are given a health boost thanks to the **hazelnuts and dates**. Hazelnuts contain a brain-stimulating combination of boron, B-complex vitamins, iron, magnesium, selenium, zinc, and omega-6 essential fatty acids. Many of these nutrients are boosted by the dates, particularly iron, magnesium, boron and B-complex vitamins, which work together to ensure healthy brain function.

4 Beat the eggs and sugar together in a large mixing bowl until light and fluffy. Then stir in the chocolate and butter mixture.
5 Sift half the flour and all the baking powder into the chocolate mixture and fold in with a wooden spoon. Sift in the remaining flour and fold in. Carefully stir in the dates and hazelnuts until evenly distributed.
6 Pour the mixture into the prepared pan and bake for 25 minutes until the brownies have risen but are still soft in the center. Leave to cool for 15 minutes before removing from the pan. Cut into 24 squares.

REAL FRUIT POPSICLES

Lower in sugar than commercially made popsicles – and certainly free from artificial coloring and other additives – these homemade popsicles are made from a real fresh fruit purée and fresh custard.

Makes 6 popsicles

6 plums, halved and pitted
3 nectarines, pitted and roughly
    chopped
1–2 tbsp unrefined superfine sugar,
    to taste
⅔ cup fresh custard

1 Put the plums and nectarines in a medium-size, nonmetallic saucepan. Add the sugar and 2 tbsp water. Bring to a boil, then reduce the heat and simmer for 5 minutes until softened. Taste for sweetness and add more sugar if too sour. Leave to cool then purée until smooth – you need about 1 cup of fruit purée.
2 Combine the fruit purée and custard, then spoon the mixture into 6 popsicle molds. Freeze until solid.

VARIATION

Orange and mango make a refreshing alternative. Juice the fruit in a juicer – you need about 1⅔ cups to make 6 popsicles. Slice 1 orange into circles and place a circle into each popsicle mold then fill with the fruit juice. Freeze until solid.

BRAIN BOX

Ice cream contains calcium, which is needed for healthy nerve function and works in tandem with magnesium to reduce irritability and insomnia.

Strawberries and oranges are rich in the potent antioxidant vitamin C, which also helps to balance the brain's neurotransmitters, having an uplifting effect.

STRAWBERRY SUNDAE

You can't go wrong with an ice cream sundae: this firm kids' favorite is a breeze to make and has been adapted to ensure a healthy twist.

Serves 4
1 pint strawberries, halved
2 tbsp fresh orange juice
1 tbsp unrefined superfine sugar
1 tbsp slivered almonds or chopped nuts
8 scoops good-quality vanilla ice cream
chocolate shavings, to serve

1 Put the strawberries and orange juice in a food processor or blender and purée until smooth. Sieve the mixture into a saucepan, to remove any seeds. Stir in the sugar and place the pan over medium-low heat; cook for 5 minutes until the sauce thickens. Taste for sweetness and add more sugar if necessary; leave to cool.
2 Lightly toast the slivered almonds or chopped nuts in a dry frying pan. Set aside to cool.
3 To serve, place a few spoonfuls of sauce in a sundae glass. Top with a scoop of ice cream and another spoonful of sauce. Add a final scoop of ice cream. Sprinkle the nuts over the top, then a few shavings of chocolate. Repeat to make four sundaes.

SWEET THINGS

All children love sweets, but it's important that they get the right sort of desserts, rather than the highly sugary, additive-laden ones commonly available. Here you'll find a variety of desserts with a healthy twist, guaranteed to appeal to your child's taste buds.

PANCAKES WITH BAKED BANANAS

A favorite with children, these substantial pancakes make an energizing family breakfast. Whole wheat flour will result in a denser pancake; for a lighter batter use half whole wheat and half white flour.

Serves 4
1¼ cups whole wheat flour
pinch of salt
2 tbsp rolled oats
2 tbsp unrefined superfine sugar
1 tsp baking powder
1 egg, beaten
1¼ cups buttermilk
⅔ cup milk
2 tbsp butter, melted
sunflower oil, for frying

for the baked bananas:
2 bananas
2 tbsp maple syrup

1 To make the baked bananas; preheat the oven to 350°F. Place the bananas on a baking sheet and bake

BRAIN BOX

Bananas are energizing foods and are a good source of the mineral potassium, which plays a key role in nerve cell function.

BRAIN BOX

Children are susceptible to the effects of fluctuating blood sugar levels, which naturally fall overnight. **Whole grains** release their energy slowly in the body, ensuring blood sugar levels are kept steady.

for 20 minutes until tender. Leave to cool slightly before slicing.

2 Meanwhile, make the pancakes. Mix together the flour, salt, oats, sugar, and baking powder.

3 Beat together the egg, buttermilk, milk, and melted butter, then add to the flour mixture. Beat well to remove any lumps, making a thick batter.

4 Lightly oil a large heavy-based frying pan and heat. Place 2 tablespoons of batter per pancake in the hot pan – you will probably be able to cook 3 pancakes at a time. Cook each pancake for 3 minutes until the base is golden, then turn over and cook for an additional 2 minutes. Place on a plate, covered with foil, to keep warm while you make the remaining pancakes.

5 To serve, divide the pancakes between four plates, spoon over the sliced baked bananas and drizzle with maple syrup.

FRUITY SHERBET

This refreshing ice is made from an antioxidant-rich combination of mangoes and oranges. It's simple to make and helps boost the recommended daily fruit intake.

Serves 6–8
½ cup unrefined superfine sugar
1¼ cups water
2 large mangoes, peeled, pitted, and
  roughly chopped
juice of 3 oranges
1 egg white

1 Put the sugar and water in a saucepan and stir until the sugar is dissolved. Place over medium-high heat and bring to a boil, reduce the heat and simmer for 5 minutes. Leave to cool.

2 Combine the mango, orange juice, and sugar syrup in a food processor or blender and process until the fruit is puréed.

3 Pour the mixture into a freezer-proof container and freeze for 2 hours until semifrozen. Remove from the freezer and break up any ice crystals using a hand-held beater.

4 Whisk the egg white until it forms stiff peaks then fold into the semi-frozen mixture. Return to the freezer and freeze until solid.

5 Transfer the sherbet to the refrigerator to soften for 30 minutes before serving.

BRAIN BOX

B-complex vitamins, found in **bread, cream, and eggs**, are crucial for converting food into energy, which the brain requires to work efficiently and effectively. It is worth noting that the eggs in this ice cream are uncooked.

BROWN BREAD ICE CREAM

Brown bread and ice cream may sound like a strange combination but it is delicious and provides plentiful amounts of mind-stimulating energy.

Serves 6–8
2 cups whole wheat bread crumbs
scant ½ cup soft brown sugar
1⅔ cups whipping cream
2 eggs, separated
2 tbsp maple syrup

1 Preheat the oven to 325°F. Combine the bread crumbs and sugar in a bowl then spread over a baking sheet. Bake, turning occasionally, until the crumbs are a dark golden color (be careful not to burn them) and the sugar has almost dissolved – the mixture almost caramelizes. Set aside.
2 In a bowl, whip the cream to soft peaks. In a separate bowl, whisk the egg whites until they form stiff peaks. Beat together the egg yolks and maple syrup in another bowl.
3 Stir the cooled sugary bread crumbs and maple syrup mixture into the whipped cream then carefully fold in the egg whites. Spoon into a freezer-proof container and freeze for a few hours until firm. Leave to soften in the refrigerator for 20 minutes before serving.

FROZEN BANANA DESSERT

Simple desserts are often the best and this couldn't be simpler. It's healthy as well, of course.

Serves 4
4 bananas, peeled
yogurt with live and active cultures, maple syrup and nuts, to serve (optional)

1 Wrap the bananas in plastic wrap and place in the freezer. Freeze until solid, then remove the plastic wrap and process in a blender until roughly chopped. The banana ice is delicious served on its own, or can be topped with a spoonful of yogurt, a drizzle of maple syrup, and a sprinkling of lightly toasted nuts.

STRAWBERRY & VANILLA FROZEN YOGURT

Lower in fat than cream ices, yogurt makes a tangy and delicious dessert. Yogurt with live and active cultures is good for the health of the digestive system, which is vital for the efficient absorption of nutrients from food.

Serves 6–8
1 quart strawberries, halved if large
1 lb Greek-style yogurt with live and active cultures
4 tbsp powdered sugar
1 tsp natural vanilla extract

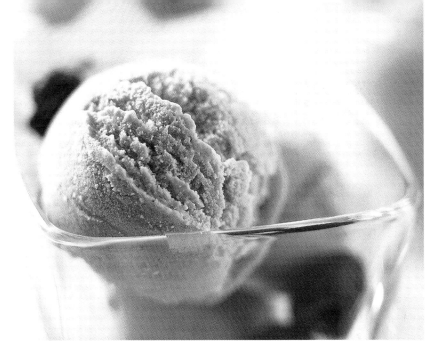

1 Preheat the oven to 400°F. Grease a 12-hole muffin pan with the extra butter or line with paper liners.
2 Mix together both types of flour with the sugar, baking powder, and salt in a mixing bowl.
3 Beat the buttermilk, eggs, and melted butter together in a separate bowl. Add the mixture to the dry ingredients and stir until just combined – there may be a few lumps but this is fine. Gently fold in the blueberries.
4 Spoon the mixture into the muffin pan and bake for 25 minutes until risen and golden.

1 Purée the strawberries in a food processor or blender until smooth. Add the yogurt, powdered sugar, and vanilla extract and process briefly to mix everything together. Pour into a freezer-proof container. (The creamy strawberry mixture is also delicious eaten as is.)
2 Freeze for 2 hours then remove from the freezer and beat by hand to break up any ice crystals that have formed. Return to the freezer for another 2 hours then repeat the beating process to break up any ice crystals. Return to the freezer again until solid.
3 Allow to soften in the refrigerator for 30 minutes before serving.

BLUEBERRY MUFFINS

The secret to good muffins is to not overmix the batter – lumps are fine, which makes them a perfect introduction to cake making for kids! A useful snack, these help to revive flagging energy levels by giving depleted blood glucose levels a boost.

Makes 16

1 stick butter, melted, plus extra
   for greasing
2¼ cups all-purpose flour
½ cup whole wheat flour
¾ cup unrefined superfine sugar
1 tsp baking powder
½ tsp salt
1¼ cups buttermilk
2 eggs, beaten
1 cup blueberries

BRAIN BOX

Blueberries are rich in powerful antioxidants called anthocyanidins. According to research, these help to mop up free radicals in both watery and fatty parts of the body, such as the brain. This is unusual in that many other antioxidants protect either the fatty or watery parts but not both.

APPLE & PLUM CRUMBLE

This fruit crumble has a crisp nutty, oaty topping. You can vary the fruit base according to what's in season – rhubarb, nectarines, berries, and pears are equally delicious. Eating apples are used here instead of cooking apples, which need plenty of sugar to sweeten them.

Serves 4–6
3 eating apples, pared, cored, and diced
squeeze of lemon juice
5 plums, halved, pitted, and diced

for the topping:
4 tbsp golden or corn syrup
6 tbsp unsalted butter
1¾ cups rolled oats
2 tbsp chopped hazelnuts
2 tbsp sunflower seeds

1 Preheat the oven to 350°F. Toss the apples in the lemon juice to prevent them from browning and arrange in a 9-inch-diameter ovenproof dish with the plums; stir well to combine.

BRAIN BOX

Apples are a good source of boron, which has been found to be important in maintaining mental alertness and concentration.

2 To make the topping, melt the syrup and butter together in a heavy-based medium-sized saucepan over medium heat. Remove from the heat and stir in the oats, hazelnuts, and seeds. Sprinkle the mixture over the top of the fruit. Bake for 20–25 minutes until golden and beginning to crisp.

DOUBLE-DECKER DATE BARS

These moist muesli-type bars contain a healthy dose of vitamins, minerals, and essential fatty acids – they're incredibly delicious too!

Makes 16 bars
1 stick butter, cubed, plus extra for greasing
1½ cups dried pitted dates, chopped
scant 1 cup water
1½ cups rolled oats
¾ cup light brown sugar
1 cup whole wheat flour
1 tsp baking powder
2 tbsp sunflower seeds
⅓ cup chopped mixed nuts

1 Preheat the oven to 350°F. Grease a 9-inch-square baking pan with the extra butter and line with parchment paper.
2 Put the dates and water in a saucepan and bring to a boil. Reduce the heat and simmer, half-covered, for 20 minutes until the dates are tender

BRAIN BOX

The brain needs a constant supply of glucose to function. Complex carbohydrates, supplied by the **whole wheat flour** and **oats** in this recipe, are the primary source of the brain's energy and also provide many nutrients.

and mushy – most of the water should have been absorbed. Purée in a blender and set aside to cool.
3 Meanwhile, mix together the oats, sugar, flour, baking powder, seeds, and chopped nuts in a large mixing bowl. Mix in the butter using your fingertips until the mixture is soft and crumbly.
4 Spoon three-quarters of the mixture into the prepared tin and press down with your fingers to make a firm, even layer. Spoon the date mixture over the oats. Sprinkle with the rest of the oat mixture and press down lightly.
5 Bake for 25 minutes until golden, then leave in the pan for 15 minutes to cool and firm up. Cut into 16 bars and remove from the pan.

MINI FRUIT CRUMBLES

These pretty, individual crumbles are perfect if you are just cooking for the children and want to make a small number of portions. They feature a nutritious combination of nectarines, oats, and seeds. Don't use overripe fruit since it will collapse during cooking.

Serves 4
4 tbsp unsalted butter, plus extra for greasing
4 nectarines, halved and pitted
¾ cup whole wheat flour
2 tbsp rolled oats
1 tbsp sunflower seeds
4 tbsp light brown sugar

1 Preheat the oven to 350°F. Grease an ovenproof dish with the extra butter. Arrange the nectarines in the dish. Add a little water to the dish to prevent the fruit becoming dry.
2 Rub together the butter and flour with your fingertips until it forms coarse bread crumbs. Stir in the oats, seeds, and sugar then mix well.
3 Spoon the crumble mixture over the nectarine halves. Bake for 20 minutes or until the crumble is golden and slightly crisp.

OATMEAL COOKIES

These cookies are packed with nutritious oats, which help to steady blood sugar levels, controlling mood swings and providing sustained amounts of energy – what more could you ask for!

Makes 10
1 stick unsalted butter
½ cup light brown sugar
⅓ cup all-purpose flour
¼ cup whole wheat flour
½ tsp baking powder
1¼ cups rolled oats

1 Preheat the oven to 350°F. Line two baking sheets with parchment paper.
2 Beat together the butter and sugar in a mixing bowl until light and fluffy. Stir in both types of flour and the oats then mix well to make a soft dough.
3 Divide the dough into 10 pieces. Roll each piece into a ball and arrange on the baking sheets, well spaced out to allow room for the cookies to spread. Flatten the top of each ball slightly and bake for 15–20 minutes until just golden but still soft in the center.
4 Leave to cool for 5 minutes then transfer to a wire rack until firm and cool.

STRAWBERRY HAZELNUT SHORTBREADS

These melt-in-the-mouth shortbreads are topped with vanilla cream and juicy strawberries in this pretty dessert. You can store any leftover shortbreads in an airtight container.

Serves 6
¾ cup all-purpose flour
½ cup whole wheat flour
¼ cup milled oats
1 tsp baking powder
pinch of salt
1 stick unsalted butter
4 tbsp unrefined superfine sugar
scant ½ cup finely chopped hazelnuts
1 tbsp milk

to serve:
½ cup heavy or whipping cream
1 tsp powdered sugar
1 tsp natural vanilla extract
strawberries, halved if large

1 Preheat the oven to 350°F. Line two baking sheets with parchment paper.
2 Combine the two types of flour with the oats, baking powder, and salt in a large mixing bowl. Rub in the butter using your fingertips until the mixture resembles fine bread crumbs. Stir in the sugar and chopped hazelnuts and mix in the milk to form a soft dough.
3 Gently knead the dough into a ball and roll out on a lightly floured work surface. Using a 2-inch cookie cutter, stamp out 12 circles and arrange on the baking sheets, spaced well apart to allow the dough to spread.
4 Bake for 15 minutes until golden but still soft in the center. Leave to cool for 5 minutes then transfer to a wire rack to cool.
5 When the shortbread is cool and you are ready to serve, whip the cream with the powdered sugar and vanilla extract until thickened. Place a shortbread on each serving plate, top with a good dollop of cream, and arrange a few strawberries on top.

BRAIN BOX

Protein foods, like **hazelnuts and dairy products**, are vital for building the brain's neurotransmitters, or messengers.

MERRY BERRY COBBLER

Berries are rich in antioxidants and vitamin C, vital for protecting the brain. Here, they are used as a base for a warming dessert that has a melt-in-the-mouth biscuit topping.

Serves 4
2 cups mixed berries, such as raspberries, blackberries, blueberries, strawberries, defrosted if frozen
8 plums, halved, pitted, and chopped
1 tsp cornstarch
3 tbsp unrefined superfine sugar

for the topping:
1 stick unsalted butter
2 tbsp unrefined superfine sugar
1¾ cups all-purpose flour
2 tsp baking powder
2 tsp cornstarch
1–2 tbsp light cream
light brown sugar, for sprinkling (optional)

1 Preheat the oven to 350°F. To prepare the fruit, put the berries and plums in an 8- x 10-inch dish. Mix the cornstarch with a little water and add to the fruit with the sugar, stir until thoroughly combined.
2 To make the topping, beat the butter and sugar together until pale and fluffy. Mix in the flour, baking powder, and cornstarch. As the mixture becomes dry, stir in the cream to form a smooth soft dough.

BRAIN BOX

This cobbler contains a healthy dose of antioxidants, including the powerful anthocyanidins found particularly in **berries**. Antioxidants are vital for protecting the brain against unwanted toxins and free radicals.

3 Divide the dough into 8 balls, flatten each one slightly and arrange on top of the berry mixture. Sprinkle lightly with light brown sugar and bake for 20–25 minutes until the top is risen and golden.

BRAIN-BUSTING GINGERBREAD!

This rich cake improves with age, becoming deliciously sticky and gooey. Molasses is much forgotten in baking, but is packed with beneficial minerals.

Makes 20 squares
1⅓ sticks unsalted butter, plus extra
    for greasing
3 cups all-purpose flour
1 cup whole wheat flour
2 tsp baking powder
1 tsp salt
3 tsp ground ginger
1 tsp baking soda
½ cup dried pitted dates, chopped
generous 1 cup milk
1 egg, beaten
1 cup light brown sugar
⅓ cup molasses
½ cup golden or corn syrup

1 Preheat the oven to 350°F. Grease an 8-inch-square cake pan with the extra butter and line the base with parchment paper.
2 Sift both types of flour, the baking powder, and salt into a large mixing bowl. Stir in the ginger, baking soda, and dates. Beat together the milk and egg and set aside.
3 Put the sugar, molasses, syrup, and butter in a saucepan, and heat, stirring, over medium-low heat until melted. Pour the mixture into the dry ingredients with the milk and egg then beat until smooth.

4 Pour the mixture into the cake pan. Level the top with the back of a spoon and bake for 55–60 minutes until a toothpick inserted into the center comes out clean. Leave the cake in the pan for 10 minutes, then turn out onto a wire rack to cool completely. Peel off the parchment paper.

BRAIN BOX

Just one tablespoon of **molasses** contains more calcium than a glass of milk, plus plenty of iron, all the B vitamins, magnesium, and manganese – it really is a super brain food. This thick, almost black syrup can be found in most supermarkets.

NUTTY APPLE CRUNCH

Another speedy low-fat version of crumble, this healthy hazelnut-topped apple purée is delicious hot or cold.

Serves 4
8 eating apples, pared, cored, and
   roughly diced

for the topping:
2 slices whole wheat bread, crusts
   removed
2 tbsp unsalted butter
⅓ cup chopped toasted hazelnuts
3 tbsp light brown sugar
1 tsp ground cinnamon

1 Process the bread in a food processor to make bread crumbs. Melt the butter in a frying pan and add the bread crumbs, hazelnuts, and sugar and cook, stirring frequently, for 3 minutes or until golden and crisp. Stir in the cinnamon and set aside.
2 Meanwhile, place the apples in a nonmetallic saucepan with 2 tablespoons of water. Cook, half-covered, over medium-low heat for 10 minutes or until very tender. Mash with a fork to break down the apples to a rough purée.
3 Sprinkle some of the hazelnut mixture into the bottom of 4 dishes, top with the apple and then the rest of the hazelnut mixture. Serve at once.

MINI PEACH TARTS

Fantastically simple, these attractive little tarts can be filled with the fruit of your choice – apples, pears, blackberries, and nectarines all work well – and they are a good way of encouraging little ones to eat more of the fresh stuff.

Makes 6
3 ripe peaches
13 oz ready-rolled puff pastry
1 egg, separated
6 tbsp fresh custard
1 tbsp unrefined superfine sugar, for
   sprinkling

1 Preheat the oven to 400°F. Line a large baking sheet with parchment paper.
2 Put the peaches in a large bowl, cover with boiling water and leave for 30 seconds. Remove from the water with a slotted spoon and, when cool enough to handle, peel off the skins. Cut each peach into quarters and remove the pit, then slice.
3 Lay out the pastry and cut six 3¼-inc-diameter circles. Arrange the pastry circles on the baking sheet and brush with egg white. Spoon 1 tablespoon of custard in the center of each pastry circle, leaving a ¾-inch border.

BRAIN BOX

The brain-protecting antioxidants vitamin C and beta-carotene are provided by the **peaches** in this dessert.

4 Fold up the edges of the pastry to encase the custard and brush the pastry with the egg yolk. Arrange the slices of peach on top of the custard and sprinkle with a little sugar. Bake for 15 minutes until the pastry is risen and golden.

MANGO FOOL

"Fool" is perhaps the wrong name for this creamy dessert, since its vitamin and mineral content can actually aid mental clarity and alertness.

Serves 4
1 large mango, peeled, pitted, and roughly chopped
scant 1 cup whipping cream
2 tsp unrefined powdered sugar
4 tbsp yogurt with live and active cultures

1 Place the mango in a food processor or blender, reserving four slices for decoration. Purée the mango until smooth.
2 Add the cream, sugar, and yogurt and blend until combined.
3 Spoon the mixture into 4 glasses and refrigerate for 1 hour to firm up slightly. Decorate each glass with a mango slice before serving.

BRAIN BOX

Although **cream** should be treated as a special occasion food and therefore not eaten every day because of its high fat content, it does provide essential protein, calcium, tryptophan, and B-complex vitamins.

LEMON PUDDING CAKES

Intensely lemony, these puddings develop a light sponge topping and a curdlike sauce at the bottom during baking. Citrus fruits are often waxed, which acts as a preservative, so make sure you buy unwaxed fruit or, if you can't find unwaxed fruit, scrub the skins with dish-washing liquid and rinse well.

Makes 6
4 tbsp unsalted butter, plus extra for greasing
scant ½ cup unrefined superfine sugar
finely grated zest and juice of 2 unwaxed lemons
3 eggs, separated
scant ½ cup milk
scant ½ cup all-purpose flour
½ tsp baking powder
pinch of salt

1 Preheat the oven to 350°F. Lightly grease 6 ramekins with the extra butter.
2 Using a handheld or electric mixer, beat together the butter and sugar until pale and smooth. Gradually beat in the lemon zest and juice – the mixture will look curdled but this is not a problem. Beat in the egg yolks, one at a time then stir in the milk, flour, baking powder and salt.
3 Whisk the egg whites in a clean, grease-free bowl until soft peaks form. Fold the egg whites into the lemon mixture until evenly incorporated. Pour the mixture into the ramekins and place the ramekins in a baking pan.
4 Pour enough hot water into the baking pan to come halfway up the sides of the ramekins and bake for 25 minutes or until the pudding cakes have risen and the tops are golden.

BRAIN BOX

Iron is found in useful amounts in **eggs**. This mineral is crucial for healthy brain function, and a lack of iron has been linked to poor concentration and depression.

PEAR BATTER PUDDING

This light dessert is similar to clafoutis, the French batter pudding, and is especially delicious served warm.

Serves 4–6
butter, for greasing
6 tbsp unrefined superfine sugar
2 ripe pears, pared, cored, and sliced
juice of ½ lemon
4 free-range eggs
1¼ cups light cream
1¼ cups full-fat milk
pinch of salt
½ cup all-purpose flour

1 Preheat the oven to 400°F. Lightly grease an 8-inch-diameter baking or gratin dish and sprinkle the base with 1 tablespoon of the sugar.

2 Dip the sliced pears in the lemon juice to prevent them browning and arrange them in the dish.

3 Put the eggs, cream, milk, salt, flour, and remaining sugar in a food processor and process until smooth and frothy. Pour this over the pears.

4 Bake for 30–35 minutes, until golden – the batter should still be quite wobbly, but it will firm up as it cools. Serve warm.

VARIATION

To make clafoutis, the classic version of this dessert, replace the pears with 20 fresh ripe pitted cherries. For other variations, you could replace the pears with 2 eating apples, pared, cored and sliced, or 4 plums, halved and pitted, or 2 peaches, pitted and sliced.

BRAIN BOX

Calcium and B-complex vitamins are found in plentiful amounts in **milk and dairy products** in general. They also contain tryptophan, which is said to aid the production of serotonin in the brain, a calming and mood-lifting chemical.

DELICIOUS DRINKS

Hydration is just as important for concentration and clarity of thought as food. Easy to make, these drinks are great alternatives to store-bought high-sugar drinks – and they are tasty, too!

MANGO & BANANA SMOOTHIE

Taste the tropics with this energy-boosting thick smoothie. Nectarines, peaches, or plums make flavorful alternatives.

Serves 3–4
1 large mango, peeled, pitted, and roughly chopped
2–3 ripe bananas, sliced
½ cup yogurt with live and active cultures
1 cup milk

1 Place the mango, bananas, yogurt, and milk in a food processor or blender and process until smooth and creamy.

BANANARAMA

Filling and substantial – the perfect protein-boosting drink to fight flagging energy levels. Serve alongside whole wheat toast or an English muffin.

Serves 2
2 ripe bananas, thickly sliced
1 tbsp smooth peanut butter
½ cup yogurt with live and active cultures
1¼ cups milk
½ tsp ground cinnamon

1 Place the bananas, peanut butter, yogurt, milk, and cinnamon in a blender. Process until smooth, thick, and frothy.

PEACH MELBA SMOOTHIE

A liquid version of the classic dessert, which provides plentiful amounts of vitamins and minerals as well as mind-stimulating protein.

Serves 2–3
3 peaches, peeled, pitted, and roughly chopped
1 generous cup raspberries
2 cups milk
3 decent scoops of good-quality vanilla ice cream

1 Place the peaches, raspberries, milk, and ice cream in a food processor or blender and process until smooth.

SUPER JUICE

Kids who start the day with this nutrient-rich juice as part of their breakfast will give their memory and energy levels a vital boost. If served with eggs, the vitamin C in the juice will aid the absorption of iron found in the eggs.

Serves 4
1 small mango, peeled, pitted, and
   roughly chopped
1 small pineapple, peeled, cored, and
   roughly chopped
1$\frac{2}{3}$ cups freshly squeezed orange juice

1 Put the mango and pineapple through a juicer or blender and combine with the fresh orange juice. Serve immediately to ensure minimum loss of vitamins, which are depleted when cut fruit is exposed to the air.

POWER JUICE

Freshly squeezed fruit and vegetable combinations are an excellent way of encouraging children to eat up their veggies and give them a vitamin boost at the same time.

Serves 2
4 apples, pared and cored
2 large carrots, peeled
handful seedless grapes

1 Put the apples, carrots, and grapes through a juicer or blender. Taste and dilute with a little water if too strong, then divide between 2 glasses and serve immediately.

ORANGE FIZZ

Ditch the sugar- and caffeine-laden carbonated drinks for this refreshing citrus vitamin C-rich alternative.

Serves 4
4 oranges
2 tbsp lemon juice
carbonated mineral water

1 Squeeze the oranges. Combine the orange juice and lemon juice in a jug and divide between four glasses. Top up with carbonated water before serving.

COCONUT & MANGO SMOOTHIE

This smoothie is similar to an Indian sweet lassi and is surprisingly filling. It is a perfect summer drink.

Serves 4

1 large mango, peeled, pitted, and chopped
14-oz can coconut milk
1 cup Greek-style yogurt
½ cup milk
2 tbsp soft light brown sugar
1 tsp ground cinnamon

1 Place the mango, coconut milk, yogurt, milk, sugar, and half the cinnamon in a food processor or blender. Process until smooth and frothy. Pour into 4 glasses and add a few ice cubes. Sprinkle with the remaining cinnamon just before serving.

VARIATION

Replace the mango with 1 large ripe banana for an equally delicious smoothie.

BRAIN BOX

Yogurt is a good source of the amino acid tyrosine, which is converted in the brain to noradrenaline and has the effect of increasing motivation and alertness. It also provides beneficial amounts of the calming magnesium, calcium, and B-complex vitamins.

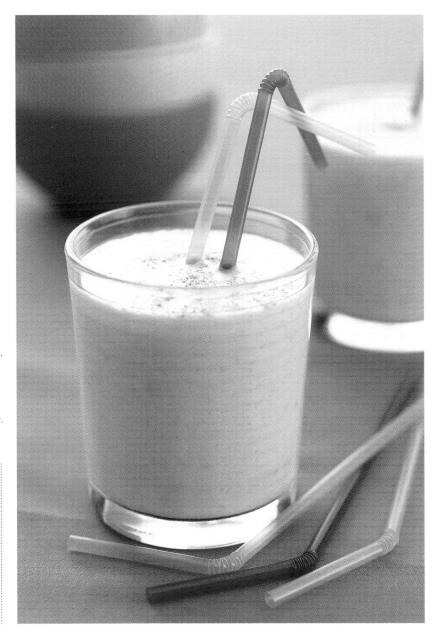

LEMON BARLEY WATER

A English child's classic, this drink does contain some sugar, but in much lower amounts than the store-bought versions. What's more, it's richer in vitamin C. Make sure you use unwaxed lemons since citrus fruit are commonly waxed, which acts as a preservative.

About 10 servings
1 cup pearl barley
2 quarts water
grated rind of 1 unwaxed lemon
juice of 3 lemons
1¼ cups unrefined superfine sugar

1 Rinse the pearl barley under cold running water then place in a large saucepan. Cover with the water and bring to a boil. Reduce the heat and simmer gently for 20 minutes, skimming off any froth that rises to the surface. Remove the pan from the heat.
2 Add the lemon rind and sugar to the pan, stir well until the sugar has dissolved and leave to cool. Strain, discarding the pearl barley, and add the lemon juice to the liquid.
3 Taste for sweetness and add more sugar if necessary. Chill before serving.

STRAWBERRIES & CREAM SMOOTHIE

This thick and creamy shake is substantial enough to make a filling breakfast if accompanied by toast. You could opt for yogurt with live and active cultures instead of vanilla ice cream, which would reduce the fat and sugar levels. Prepare just before serving for optimum nutrient levels.

Serves 3–4
1 pint strawberries, halved if large
1¼ cups milk
½ tsp pure vanilla extract
3 decent scoops of good-quality vanilla ice cream

BRAIN BOX

Milk is a complete protein, meaning that it contains all eight essential amino acids, one of which is the brain-stimulating tyrosine.

Strawberries are a good source of vitamin C, carotenoids, and some B-complex vitamins.

1 Place the strawberries in a food processor or blender and process until puréed. Add the milk, vanilla, and ice cream and process until thick and creamy.

HONEY BERRY FIZZ

This low-sugar version of a popular fruit drink can be diluted with still or carbonated water but the latter always goes down well. The bags of frozen mixed red berries you can buy in supermarkets are ideal for this.

Serves 4

7 oz frozen fruit, including a mixture of fruit such as blackberries, raspberries, and strawberries
2 tbsp honey
carbonated or still water, to serve

1 Place the berries and honey in a saucepan and gently heat through, stirring occasionally, until the fruit has defrosted and is very juicy. Transfer to a blender and process until fairly smooth.
2 To remove any seeds in the fruit, press the mixture through a sieve into a bowl and discard the pulp and seeds. Pour the juice into a jug. Leave to cool then refrigerate, covered, until ready to serve. To serve, half fill a glass with the berry juice and top with water.

BRAIN BOX

Dehydration can affect behavior, leading to poor concentration, tiredness, and depression. It is vital for children to drink enough **fluids** throughout the day to help with mental energy.

BRAIN BOX

The calcium and magnesium found in **milk** are known as nature's tranquilizers, which is why they make such good bedtime drinks.

Almonds are also rich in these minerals as well as memory-boosting B vitamins, omega-6 essential fatty acids, and zinc.

USE-YOUR-NUT SHAKE

A hint of chocolate adds to the popularity of this wholesome frothy milk shake.

Serves 2

6 tbsp slivered almonds
2 ripe bananas, thickly sliced
1¼ cups milk
2 tbsp good-quality chocolate drink powder

1 Grind the almonds in a blender until finely ground and smooth. Add the bananas, milk, and chocolate powder then blend until smooth and frothy.

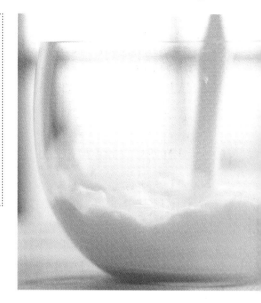

REAL HOT CHOCOLATE

A real calming treat at the end of the day – why use powdered cocoa when you can enjoy the real thing?

Serves 1

1 cup milk
¾–1 oz bittersweet chocolate, broken (plus grated chocolate to decorate)
½ tsp maple syrup

1 Gently heat the milk in a small saucepan.
2 Break the chocolate into the milk and whisk until the chocolate has melted and the milk is frothy.
3 Pour into a mug and stir in the maple syrup. Decorate with a little grated chocolate and serve.